Suicidal Children and Adolescents

Other books by the same author

Cotton Everywhere (1994) Aurora Press
A Thanatology of the Child (1998) Mark Allen Publishing Limited
A Northern Thanatology (1998) Mark Allen Publishing Limited
A Thanatology of War (1998) Mark Allen Publishing Limited

Suicidal Children and Adolescents

Christine Kenny

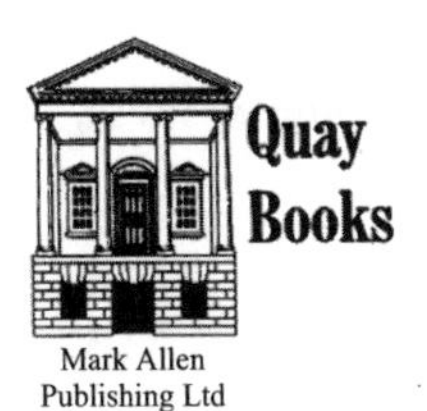

Quay Books Division, Mark Allen Publishing Limited,
Jesses Farm, Snow Hill, Dinton, Wiltshire, SP3 5HN

British Library Cataloguing-in-Publication Data
A catalogue record is available for this book

ISBN 1 85642 132 5

Printed in the UK by The Cromwell Press, Trowbridge, Wiltshire

Contents

Acknowledgements

I would like to thank my parents, Joan and Ben Miller, Bill Kenny and Colin Purcell-Lee, and my children Lisa, Mark, Leonard and Philip for all their support during the time that I have spent researching and writing this book and for their comments and help with the proof reading. Thanks also to Vic Finkelstein, Jeremy Weinstein, Pittu Laungani, Sally and Richard Skillett-Moore, Joe Greenwood, Laura Markowe, David McLoughlin, Peter Davis, Tony Walter and Laverne Pearson.

Introduction

Crisis and confusion in a post-modern world

It seems that there has never been a more difficult time to write about subjects that hinge on the importance of definitions. One of the more negative consequences of the impact of post-modernity, is that the assumptions, classifications, theories and definitions on which social science has depended, have been challenged, scrutinised and deconstructed.[1] Indeed, in relation to concepts such as 'social class', definitions appear to have turned back on themselves. The (former) middle-class are now the working-class. The former working-class, the underclass. The former middle class, some of them social scientists, who may have identified with the capitalist, the 'upper-class', suddenly find that the finger of the factory clock is pointing at them. It wants their time.[2] And in exchange for their labour, it expects value for money. It is little wonder that the world appears 'upside down' and 'back to front'. Do these comments suggest a little working-class 'smugness'? If so, then let me assure the reader that this is really not the case. After all, given my education, I suppose I am now considered middle-class. I am also a social scientist. The finger of the factory clock is pointing at me. These are comments on observed realities and are not meant to be humorous, particularly when we relate them to rising suicide rates among children and adolescents. Scientific and technological advances have brought benefits, but they have costs, one of which is unemployment. The intentions behind most inventions are usually benevolent. The idea is to do good. Let us not forget that Dr Frankenstein was destroyed by the monster he created, and not without the loss of a few 'innocent' casualties.

1 Despite the apparent elusiveness of any fixed, dependable definitions for the period that has become known as post-modernism, numerous attempts have been made, though somehow (in the writer's experience) these almost always move into discussions of what it is not, rather than what it is. Nettleton (1995, p.34) for example, identifies three 'not ifs' in her discussion, and refers the reader to the work of Featherstone (1991) and Smart (1992) for a more detailed discussion.

2 And in doing so, developed theory after theory that pathologised oppressed groups and their strategies for resistance.

Definitional problems have always been a characteristic of complex phenomena, such as childhood, adolescence, mental health and suicides, even when we narrow our investigation down to the analysis of isolated variables. Such enquiries become even more challenging when we try to visualise the various systems that govern their interaction. One of the strengths of 'grand theory' is that the patterns it weaves (or at least appears to weave) have some coherence. They tell a convincing story. Now these grand theories have been deconstructed.[3] We are left with a box of confusing, unravelled threads and little else to work with beyond a universe of discourse. Everything is 'relative', 'socially constructed'. To take a moral position on almost anything in this context, leaves one open to charges of racism, sexism, class discrimination, disableism; the list is endless. Buzz terms such as 'non interference' serve as euphemisms for 'sod off and leave me alone. I can't be bothered'. The result is, at best, the search for new and interesting alternatives, at worst, intellectual paralysis.[4]

Do academic trends reflect rather than create the consequential insecurities of post-modernity?[5] The author assumes the former to be the case. The realities amount to more than abstractions. The world has become more diverse, fragmented and uncertain. The challenge to authority, such as that of the 'scientist', may have broken down hierarchies, consequentially allowing for more (apparently) equitable relationships. But it has also led to insecurities. The 'truths' spawned from the mouths of 'experts' have certain advantages. They can be comforting when you are ill, or when you are searching for 'solid' dependable predictions. Reliable advice from child care experts offers dependable strategies to help timid new parents cope. An oral history of northern working-class women's experience revealed that access to the health clinic and health visitor was one of the benefits most welcomed by these women when the NHS came into being (Kenny, 1994). At a time when access to experts is increasingly limited (due to the gradual rolling back of the Welfare State) parents are expected to shoulder more and more responsibility. In the public sector, never before has so much time been devoted to writing and

3 Especially those which are scientifically based, eg. attacks on crude interpretations of post-modernism, the author would argue, have the potential to seriously undermine the validity of any positive contributions that may have been made.

4 Most significant (and increasingly so as academia becomes increasingly proletarianised) is that even the expert is losing faith in the expert. Note the vast amount of literature in which writers happily engage in discussion of what is not, but 'shy' away from discussions of what is.

5 Question raised during an informal conversation with colleagues, 1998.

talking about 'quality'. And never before has there been so little time given to the practice of actually delivering it. Young people, children and new parents struggle in a context of hesitancy. Taking a life-span approach, there was once a time when 'grand theories' postulated that childhood instability could pose threats to mental health in later life. Now these grand theories arc in themselves 'unstable'. What will be the long-term consequences of living in a post-modern world?

Post-modernity is a term used to describe realities of change that pose threats to identity. These are due to 'an interaction between economic and cultural factors whereby changes in production and consumption patterns can be seen as producing new shared identities' (Woodward, 1997). Globalisation has caused the dissolution and dispersal of older, established communities based on geographic location through the mass migration of labour that 'produces identities which are shaped and located in many different places. These new identities can be both settling and unsettling' (Woodward, *op cit*). Conversely, 'post-modernism' can be (and is perhaps too often) interpreted as a denial of these or, indeed, any external realities. One of the most powerful assumptions underpinning psychological theories of personality was the concept of a 'core self'. Even this has been challenged and deconstructed (Giddens, 1991), but not yet reconstructed. 'Self' is no longer 'what we are' but rather 'what we do' and 'how we spend'. Compared to authenticity, consumerism presents 'dicey' foundations on which to build a positive sense of self. Any such construction can only last (only begin) as long as the 'dosh' is coming in. But what is the best way to ensure that it does come in. A participant who took part in this study summarised the dilemmas that young people are faced with:

> I feel down when I'm skint, but that's not a major thing cos I know that will pass. Well, I hope it will! Being bored, out of a job and not feeling that I'm doing much with my life. Not knowing what I'd like to do. It seems that there are not that many chances these days to better yourself. Then, when you think about it you get tired, it seems too much sometimes. I'd like to get some more education but then I'd need some money. So I think, 'well I need to get a job first'. Then I realise that, to get a really good job I need an education. Its hard knowing which direction to turn really. You seem to be blocked at every turn, like, if you try to get an education while you are signing on, well you lose benefits. And most of the jobs that are advertised around here, well the wages are so bad that you would have to work all the hours God sent to make a wage that you could live

> on. So that cuts out getting an education while you work. But then, even if you get an education, there's no jobs. I think its really hard.[6]

At a time when unemployment is rising, especially in the young (at the very time when they are striving to establish an identity) this is worrying. Western society is suspended in a period that is unnameable, lacking clearly defined and articulated characteristics. This is a period more concerned with defining not what is, but rather, what is not. A period more concerned with understanding the meaning assigned to phenomena, than in any attempt to provide explanation for what might have contributed to the creation of that phenomena. As Nettleton (1995) suggests, 'it could be argued that the need, or search for, absolute truths has become a spurious exercise within a post-modern society'. The search for truth which was grounded in rational science is a fundamentally modernist project. This can make the world appear very confusing. A crude interpretation could allow us to believe that all that is, is merely a construction, an illusion, a relativity.[7] The goal is to deconstruct, to expose the assumptions that form the basis of scientific enquiry. Given that assumptions are the basis of all thought (where are you coming from?) such attention is important. This has led to an important shift, to the creation of new starting points, the formulation of new questions and in endeavouring to answer them, new solutions or 'stories'. As Frosh (1991) explains in his discussion of 'Post-modern states of mind':

> *The image of modernity presented above evokes a world in which survival is constantly threatened by startling forces which have the power to turn everything upside down and to destroy those precious achievements of personal integrity and interpersonal affection towards which people strive. At the same time, it claims the dizzying kaleidoscope of modern experience provides individuals with opportunities for development of their own capacities for representation and construction.*

Living in a post-modern world implies both threats to and potentiality for the formation and maintenance of identities. In such a context,

6 20-year-old unemployed male.

7 Even the validity of the term 'post-modernism' has been challenged. Nettleton (1995) for example, acknowledges that whereas some argue that post-modernism is a new social form, others consider it to be an intensification of the features of modernity; in other words, modernity in the extreme. On this basis some writers prefer the term 'high modernity' rather than 'post-modernity'.

security, trust, intimacy, all of the things that we assume provide 'buffers' to shield the individual against alienation and stress become problematic. How do we know for sure that they exist, let alone how to search for and establish them. Giddens (1991) explores the relationship between trust, identity and risk. He argues that, 'in circumstances of uncertainty and multiple choice, the notions of trust and risk have particular application'. Like Erikson (1950) he considers trust to be one of the most fundamental building blocks on which personality is built. Once established between caretaker and child, it provides an 'inoculation' that screens off potential threats and dangers that, 'even the most mundane activities of day-to-day life contain'. The establishment of trust is essential to avoid what he describes as a 'paralysis of will' that would inhibit the 'leap into faith' that is a necessary part of all social interaction. Relating his discussion to the uncertainties of post-modernity, he continues, 'doubt, a pervasive feature of modern critical reason, permeates into everyday life as well'. What do theoretical discussions such as this have to do with the realities of life that the young people represented in this study have to contend with? What does depression and suicide have to do with young people? A very great deal as it may be the very pervasiveness of this lack of certainty and confidence that contributes to young people's unhappiness.

This book addresses the issue of suicidal children and young people. *Chapter 1* considers some of the factors that contribute to suicide in young children, beginning with a discussion of informed intent, ie. exploring the question of whether young children, given that they have immature understandings of death, are intellectually capable of committing suicide. Children's cognitive, emotional and social development in relation to death, depression and the development of suicidal thoughts are explored, as are lifespan approaches, drawing specifically on Erikson's (1950) emphasis on the importance of the development of trust and discussing the implications that this has for mental health in the child and later life. The chapter ends with the conclusion that children can and do make informed choices when they attempt or commit suicide. However, the meaning that motivates the act (and indeed the meaning that the child wishes to convey) is probably very different from an adult. *Chapter 2* addresses the issue of adolescent suicide. Again, some of the variables that might contribute to suicide are explored, including conflicts due to separation and identity. Leenaars (1995) refers to suicide prevention, intervention and post-intervention. Prevention refers to the promotion of mental well-being and the prevention of suicide. This is discussed in *Chapter 3*. Post-intervention refers to support for survivors following a completed suicide. *Chapter 4* considers the experiences of those bereaved by suicide and the various forms of support that are available. The *Appendix* provides a summary of some of the organisations that exist to support young people in times of crisis bereavement.

The work has evolved from a series of in-depth interviews with 19 men and 12 women aged between 18 to 60 years of age, living in the north west of England, London and the Midlands. Some of the participants had considered suicide at some time in their lives. Others had suffered bereavements due to a suicide. Five of the participants had encountered suicide directly or indirectly in the course of their work. Other participants had no experience of suicide whatsoever, but were willing to offer opinions. Given the emotive and painful subject of the investigation, every attempt was made to make the data gathering process as informal as possible. Some flexibility in approach was required because many of the participants, although willing to take part in the study, refused to have the interviews taped. In such cases it was necessary to write notes during the interview with the unfortunate consequence that much of what has been said was lost. Research such as this implies important ethical considerations and so no children have been included in the sample. The experiences of suicide recorded are based on adult, auto-biographic memories. This produces obvious limitations for the research. Autobiographic memory differs in important ways from that of conceptual and factual memory. It has, for example, perhaps the greatest potential for inaccuracies and distortion (Conway, 1990a). However, it also has many strengths, including the ability to convey feelings and experience with greater impact (Stanley, 1994).

Gaining access to participants was an informal process, commonly referred to in the social sciences as 'snowball' sampling, ie. access to one or two participants led to recommendations and introductions to other participants. The author acknowledges that such an informal (by positivist standards) piece of research is limited as many findings can be generalised. However, the aims of qualitative research such as this is exploratory, seeking to map out themes that may be worthy of further exploration in a larger study and explore the meaning and complexity of an issue (Oakley, 1991). In this research, the concern has been to let people tell their stories, in their own way and on their own terms with minimal academic intrusion. Where necessary some identifying features have been removed.

The data has been interpreted mainly from a psychological

perspective, drawing on many of the 'grand theories' that have been recently challenged.[8] Many of these theories have been based on white, western, heterosexual, male assumptions. However, these have much to offer, perhaps most significantly because they were developed at a time when qualities, such as specialism, rigour and systematic observation counted for something. Because of this, and despite weaknesses or limitations to their work, these 'great masters' although mostly male, actually did identify some timeless, universal aspects of human experience. These qualities seem more rather than less important in the context of post-modernity. Erikson's theoretical framework, for example, has proved an invaluable base from which to explore some of the issues identified by the research and discussed in this book. It is true that traditional psychological 'grand theories' are based on western constructions of the child. This construction conveys an implicit 'truth' that the author believes in; that children and young people do not think in the way that adults think. They see the world differently from adults. Their perceptions, no matter how 'valid' from the point of view of their own perspective, are **immature** in developmental terms.

It is important, of course, to acknowledge that Erikson (1950) theorised on the basis of observations made during a different historical and social context. This has implications for how we draw on his analysis. For example, Erikson developed his theory of lifespan development at a time when certain expectations in life appeared realistic. Such expectations included the possibility of having a job for life. There was a belief that long-term planning could ensure a degree of certainty and security in life, in cause effect relationships and in the ability to be able to make predictions on the basis of having identified these. Things have changed. This book explores the issue of suicidal children and young people within the context of post-modernity, although this does not imply that post-modernism is the cause of suicide. Many of the characteristics that underpin post-modernity may contribute to it, but suicide is not, by any means, a phenomenon that can be associated solely with the present time.

8 However, the writer has drawn on some of the theories that have been developed in the field of health promotion in *Chapter 3*. These theories are extremely capable (and indeed have their base) with psychological theory and have proved very useful in making speculations based on this study, of what the implications of the research may be for the promotion of mental health and well-being in the young.

Literature review

Wass writes:

> *Youth and death! This association seems inappropriate and contradictory. Youth represents life, growth and the future. Death marks the end of growth and life.*
>
> 1995

Despite all the hope and optimism that we commonly associate with youth, there has been an alarming increase in recent years in the suicide rates of children and young people in affluent countries (Rioch, 1994; Leenaars, 1995). After accidents, suicide is currently the most common cause of death among young men between 20 and 24 years of age in this country (the Samaritans, 1998). Dominion (1990) attributes the earliest and most comprehensive study of suicide in young people to the work of Lourie (1957). This study found that some of the first official reports of suicide in young children appeared in Prussia in the late eighteenth century. In England there was a slight increase in child suicide rates at the turn of the century. This was followed by a consistent fall into the 1930s after which there has been a steady increase. Currently, in many of the more affluent countries, suicide in the young, especially young men, is increasing at an appalling rate. In Canada suicide rates for young adults are as high, if not higher, than for the elderly. A Swedish study conducted between 1955 and 1959 found that during the course of the study, 1727 suicides had been attempted by young people. The oldest was a 21-year-old, the youngest was aged ten years. Young women accounted for 80% of the recorded attempts. Young men were found to have a much higher rate of having completed suicides. A follow-up study conducted in 1960 demonstrates that suicide attempts should be taken very seriously. Of the experimental group, 84 had committed suicide compared to 24 who had done so in the control group (Otto, 1972). A study conducted between 1962 and 1968 in England and Wales, found that 31 children had committed suicide during the course of six years. It was estimated that this constituted around one child in 800,000 of the population at that time. Of these deaths, 10 had occurred in the 13-year-old group, 26 in the 14-year-old group; highlighting the fact that suicide attempts can begin quite young, around the time that children are beginning to develop what Piaget (1965) described as formal operational thinking (the ability to think in abstract ways, understanding what you are doing (Mc Clure, 1984).

In 1965, Connell suggested that the annual total of suicides in England committed by young people came to between 1204 and 1600. Recent work by the Samaritans (1998) suggests that whether or not we take intent into account, 'a large proportion of young people actually do die by their own hand'. The study estimated that suicide was the third most common cause of death in young people aged between 15 and 24 years of age. In younger people aged between 10 and 15 years, the rate was 1.7/100 000, or 330 deaths in 18 860 000 children. The results of this study are even more disturbing when we consider that the first most common cause of death was due to unintentional injuries and the second was homicide. Viewing these three causes of death collectively supports the view put forward by Wass (1995) that a great many young people in Western society are exposed to an unacceptable level of violence and neglect. It seems natural to respond to such insights with moral outrage but, in the long-term, is such a response helpful in initiating change? If we are to initiate change then we need first to understand why change is necessary.

There is no universally accepted definition of suicide and Leenaars (1995) argues it is impossible to develop one. Nevertheless, Shneidman in 1985 argued that this was essential if the relatively new discipline of suicidology was to have a conceptual basis for its subject of investigation. He defined suicide as:

> *A conscious act of self-induced annihilation, best understood as a multi-dimensional malaise in a needful individual who defines an issue for which the suicide is perceived as the best possible solution.*

Social science's interest in suicide began to emerge at the turn of the century, most notably with the work of Durkheim and Freud. Research on the subject has been beset with problems. Much has been noted about the difficulty in using official statistics due to the unwillingness of many coroners to record a verdict of suicide, particularly in the case of a child or young adult. Further, families are more likely to hide any evidence of suicide (eg. notes) if they belong to a culture or subgroup in which a strong stigma is attached to the act. Atkinson (1975), for example, notes that Catholics are more prone to hide such evidence. Despite these considerations, Wertheimer (1991) observes that suicide rates do appear to be higher in the more affluent countries. Alongside this, the methodologies employed by forensic scientists are improving, as is the accurate gathering of statistics.

Theories of what leads a person to commit suicide are countless and many reduce the enquiry to the investigation of a number of variables. In reality, suicide is a very complex phenomenon. A predisposition towards suicide usually evolves over time and the 'full' picture involves several of the following elements:

- ❖ The person may have experienced long-term, unbearable pain. Leenaars (1995) refers to the profound effects of the 'pain of feeling pain'. Such pain can be so intense that the sufferer has no means to communicate what it is like. What appear to be acts of 'manipulation', 'blackmail' or 'attention seeking' may be an attempt to communicate this pain.
- ❖ The links between suicide and unemployment are unclear, although several writers have argued strongly that such a link exists, especially in young men (Royal College of Psychiatrists, 1987). [9]
- ❖ Wass (*op cit*) asserts that older, intellectually bright, mentally healthy young people are less likely to have suicidal thoughts, although he provides no evidence to support this claim.
- ❖ Long-term disruption and disorganisation in a family has also been postulated as a contributing factor, but studies exploring this possibility have been criticised on methodological grounds.
- ❖ Whether or not there are significant gender differences in suicide intent is open to much debate. It is certainly the case that more men complete whereas more women attempt. To what degree motivation to complete may differ between the sexes is difficult to establish.
- ❖ Sometimes physical impairment (especially if it involves loss of a bodily part) or chronic illness can cause a person to feel suicidal.
- ❖ Illnesses that have implications for an individual's mental health, such as anorexia, bulimia or diabetes can leave the individual in a particularly vulnerable position (Barraclough, 1986).

Not all suicidal people are depressed and *vice versa*. The depressed person is at greater risk because a characteristic of this condition is the feeling of unbearable, unendurable pain. According to Shneidman (1985), unendurable pain (physical or psychological in origin) rather than depression is one of the greatest causes of suicide. Leenaars (*op cit*) infers that the individual wants to flee from pain, and that, 'the fear is that the trauma, the crisis, is bottomless, an eternal suffering. The person feels boxed in, rejected, deprived, forlorn, distressed, and especially hopeless and helpless'. Previous suicide attempts provide a reasonable prediction of the likelihood of further attempts, but it is important not to be too confident in making

9 *The Independent*, 20 April, 1987, cited by Wertheimer (1991).

generalisations. Some of the data collected for this book suggest that the reverse might be true (see *pp. 25*). Kobler and Stotland (1964) have shown that labelling people as 'suicidal' can significantly increase the risk of further attempts. Manninger (1938) had observed that there are important differences (as well as similarities) between attempts and those who complete an act of suicide. In cases of para (or attempted) suicide, the pain is **potentially** unendurable. As such, para suicide may sometimes constitute an attempt to reduce tension and provoke a response (Stengel, 1964). In other words, it is a cry for help. A completed suicide constitutes a solution to unendurable pain. Milligan and Clare (1993) challenge distinctions between the two phenomena, arguing that 'people who engage in repeated acts of self harm often do end up dying at their own hand, either deliberately or accidentally'. Of his own experience of depressive illness Milligan writes:

> *Only when you know what it is like to feel depressed, to feel that you are dying inside, can you know what it is like to be suicidal, to think that the whole dreadful, terrible, nagging, awful pain of it all might be swept away by a simple, single act of self destruction.*

In practical (as opposed to perceived) terms, it could be argued that the older one gets, the more roles and responsibilities one has to take on board and, the more exposed to external causes of stress one becomes. However, stress is due to the interaction of internal (perception, level of tolerance, personality variables, etc.) as well as external forces. Acknowledgement of the existence of stress does not always provide a corresponding ability to cope. Nor does perception of ability necessarily correspond with actual ability. People are surprising. Those who consider themselves cowardly or weak (or *vice versa*) often demonstrate behaviour that completely contradicts that person's self-perception. Do the findings of the study suggest that younger people, in general, perceive themselves to be more able to cope with stress (a belief that may become seriously challenged when faced with the reality)? If so, then such individuals may understandably feel less tolerant towards those who seem unable to cope with the pressures of life. Indeed, they may feel less tolerant towards themselves if confronted with the lack of an ability to cope. Alternatively, the response may suggest that younger people feel less able to admit to themselves, or to anyone else, their own vulnerability. There are numerous hallmarks to maturity, but it could be argued that one is the ability to recognise and admit to human vulnerability.

Early adolescence is considered to be a time when people are more likely to be confident, adventurous and able to take risks. It might be harder for a younger person to admit to feeling overwhelmed, especially to peers. The findings of the Samaritans' study is quite crucial in this respect, because the research highlighted that younger people are more likely to turn to a peer for help if they feel depressed, rather than to members of their own family or adults. In view of this, there appears to be a real urgency for increasing knowledge and understanding of depression in younger people. Yet 66% of the young people who took part in the Samaritans' study did not consider suicide an 'easy' way out. This indicated some sensitivity to the suffering of those who are driven to it. Despite this, a further 26% of the younger sample disagreed, suggesting a fair degree of intolerance. It would seem that age, in itself, offers only a partial insight into attitudes and beliefs towards suicide. Other variables, such as personality and perhaps direct experience, may be influential. Although comprehensive at a descriptive level, the Samaritans' study did not conduct more advanced analysis of the data, eg. cluster analysis, correlations. This might have allowed for such relationships (if and where they existed) to emerge. Twenty-nine percent of the younger sample, for example, knew of someone who had died of suicide and, within this group, 16% reported that the deceased had been an immediate family member or friend. Were these the same people who expressed a greater level of tolerance towards suicide generally, or might the reverse be the case? Does direct experience of having someone close commit suicide lead to more or less tolerance? Further research or, alternatively, a more advanced analysis of the data collected by the Samaritans, might provide answers to these questions.

1

Suicidal children

Introduction

Suicide is a deliberate, violent act. The ability to commit this act implies the potential to make informed decisions based on a complete understanding of the implications and potential consequences of performing that act. We could argue from this perspective that for an act of suicide to qualify as such, the deceased fully understood the consequences of what he/she was doing, that, for example, death is final and irreversible. Deconstruction of Western 'childhood' reveals abstractions such as 'innocence' and 'immaturity'. These contradict any acceptance that a child could commit suicide. The execution of a successful suicide requires a lot of planning, a mature degree of intelligence and a clear understanding of what it is that one hopes to achieve. It could be argued, that a mature understanding of death is required to qualify a death as an informed act. The evidence to support the view that children's understanding of death is qualitatively different from that of adults is overwhelming. This was observed by one of the funeral directors who took part in this study:

> I think that it takes guts to commit suicide, to really commit it. I mean, those who really mean to do it, you'd be amazed at the amount of planning that goes into it. That really does become very clear when you have been in the business as long as me. It's clear, when you look into the background, that they have spent weeks maybe planning it, and some of them are very smart. I mean, you actually do need to be pretty smart in many ways, to do it successfully. Some mean to do it, but they don't plan it, or didn't know how, what they were doing. That's when they can fail, but it's quite serious because they can end up really hurting themselves. But when they plan it, they'll do things like swimming around and around and around, until they're so tired they just sink. You think about it. Its actually quite hard to drown if you can swim because its an instinctive thing to swim like, if that's what you can do. So to plan a drowning when you can swim, that needs a good understanding of that kind of, instinctive drive to survive, you know, even when you don't want to. It might seem a funny thing to

> say, especially when you are talking about something that isn't very nice like that [suicide]. But it really is the case that, you are struck by how well planned many acts of suicide are. That's why I think suicide in a child is a real shame, but not possible really, not in that way. I mean, to plan something like that, you do need I would think, a certain level of intelligence and maturity. I don't think myself that a child has that. I think it's more a case of accidental death. I do think children may be unhappy, and may want to sort of, escape, or cry for help. But with the experience I've had, I find it very hard to believe that a child could plan, and sort of, make decisions like that.

The assumption underpinning many traditional developmental theories in psychology, is that children have a different perception of the world from that of adults; that they have specific emotional needs, which have to be nurtured. Human babies are completely helpless and dependant. Few might disagree that very young children need an adult caretaker to attend to their physical needs. But Aries (1960) notes that for many centuries (certainly throughout the Middle Ages and well into the fifteenth century) people believed that children were miniature adults. This concept, known as preformation theory, assumed that at conception, a fully formed human being was implanted in the uterus. Children differed from adults only in their size. As soon as a child was able to walk and talk, he or she joined in adult games, performed the same tasks and wore the same kinds of clothes (Crain, 1980). Children, like adults, were considered to be fully aware of the consequences of their actions and were held fully responsible for them. From this perspective (presumably) there would be little doubt that a child would be completely capable of committing suicide.

However, even if we accept that children do understand death differently, does a difference in understanding constitute an inability to perform an act? If this is the case, can we conclude that there exists a specific age (or stage) at which a child becomes capable of committing suicide? Prior to reaching this stage, is any death brought about by a child's own hand accidental rather than suicidal? Identification of stages requires decisions about dimensions around which to set criteria. Chronological age is a commonly used criterion that establishes the adult from non-adult. The impoverished potential this offers as a basis for analysis becomes clear when compared with criteria that are psychological in nature (Whitworth and Wienstock, 1979). The psychological dimensions of personality are extremely complex and include measures, such as perception, emotion, interpretation and intellect. For the sake of simplicity, ease of comprehension and to establish familiarity, we can set these out as separate entities (as we have in the following discussion). In reality, these are interrelated, incapable of providing explanations if taken in isolation. On this basis, should we conclude that the meaning behind such an act would be different in the case of a child? It certainly seems to be the case that children interpret such events differently. This is clear from the extract of the transcript cited below:

> A friend of mine committed suicide. I do remember he had a habit of saying, 'I wish I was dead'. We never took him seriously, we never took him on really. I remember his brother [of the deceased] coming around to our house. He was hysterical like, really, it took us ages to get it out of him what his brother had done and even then, when he told us, we couldn't really understand it. He just kept telling us that his brother was dead. We kept talking about him being dead, but we kept kind of waiting for him to come back then he could tell us why he'd done it. I remember that for weeks and weeks our parents kept having these meetings. We couldn't really understand what they were saying. We couldn't even understand it at his funeral. Some of the parents kept saying it was an accident. It was the talk around for ages, but you get different stories. We were never really sure if he committed suicide or not. But when I think of it, I think of him committing suicide to be honest. The funeral wasn't that good really, with all the adults there. They tried to be nice, but it was our mate you see? So, after a few weeks, we all met in the park. One of us had nicked some matches. We lit a little fire and we all said something nice to him like, 'don't half miss you mate'. Some of us had managed to nick some cigarettes off our parents as well [the deceased enjoyed an occasional cigarette] and we threw them in the fire and said 'here you are mate'.[1]

There are several themes in the extract above that support the assumption that children's understanding of death is different from that of adults. For example, the belief that the dead person will come back (Kitzinger and Kitzinger, 1989); that death is something that is 'done' to someone (Anthony, 1971). There is a suggestion consistent with the finding of Fitzgerald (1992) that death is perceived as a different kind of 'being alive'. From this perspective, the dead exist

1 30-year-old male participant's recollection of a friend who committed suicide or died accidentally (the cause was never legally established according to this participant).

living in a different but somehow parallel dimension, in which access to gifts such as cigarettes seems a realistic goal.[2] Despite any efforts of adults to support the children, the participant recalls that he and his friends needed to have their own meetings and discussions. The adults were excluded. This suggests that children do, to an extent, live in a different conceptual world. It is observations such as this that led Kubler-Ross (1983) to the conclusion that children share a 'special' symbolic language. However, it is also clear from the account that the young man had received inconsistent stories and explanations. The case continued to have an air of secrecy about it, despite attempts on the part of adults to be open and supportive. Indeed, even in adulthood, the young man is unable to say for sure whether it is suicide or an accidental death that he recalls. This was a common feature in all the stories of child suicide gathered for this study. Death is difficult enough for parents to explain to children. Explaining an act of suicide, especially if committed by a peer, is even more difficult but perhaps desirable. It seems from the extract above that the secrecy (and possible fear and embarrassment) that surrounded the case, made it much more difficult for peers of the deceased to understand what had happened. It is equally clear that the young people had a strong need to make some sense of what had happened. A need so great that when the parents failed to provide some way of doing this, the young people set out to find some way to assign meaning themselves. Would they have engaged in the ritual described above, regardless of any support or explanations provided by adults.

Suicide, especially if committed by a child, challenges our moral and value assumptions. Such actions present a serious challenge to dominant notions of the 'innocence' of the child. For all these reasons and many more, we have to accept that statistical evidence gives us only a partial insight into the complexity and gravity of the problem. We must consider the reluctance of coroners to record a verdict of suicide, especially if the evidence they are presented with conflicts with 'common sense' assumptions about what initiates or constitutes such an act. Many suicides fail to be certified as such, especially if the case involves the death of a child (Atkinson, 1975;

2 This participant is describing the behaviour of 10- to 11-year-olds. Some of the themes identified in this narrative are more consistent with what one might expect in much younger children (aged around four to six years of age). Other themes are completely consistent with the age group discussed. This suggests that children's understanding of death can operate at several different levels at the same time. Perhaps emotion (eg. regression) can account for this?

Leenaars, 1995). Problems are understandable when we consider the child's position in law. The law officially denies the possibility of clear criminal intent in children under a certain age. Prior to this, children are not considered responsible for their own actions. If children are unable to understand the nature and full implications of a criminal act, then it is equally possible that they are incapable of suicide.[3] But is this necessarily accurate, or helpful? Such assumptions lead to inaccurate recording, making statistics unreliable. It can also encourage a tendency to underestimate the seriousness of emotional problems when they are observed in young people. Another participant recalled:

> When I was a child, a child, a 13-year-old lad that I was at school with... to be honest... I can't remember that much about it because it was sort of masked over. We were just told that he had died, and then we heard rumours that he had taken too many tablets, although no one actually admitted that he'd committed suicide, even though a week or two before his death, two suicide notes had been found in his desk. Well, not suicide notes as such, but notes saying how unhappy he was, like, looking back that did indicate that he might be at risk. But no one took any notice of them. To be honest, he was a bit of a loner. None of us were that close to him, well he didn't really seem that interested in making friends. I suppose, some people thought he might be a bit 'snooty' though, looking back, he might just have been shy. You see things differently don't you, when you're older. I think some of the kids bullied him, but being a loner, you never knew for sure. I think the whole thing was handled very badly to be honest, before and after. I mean, had we understood him a little better, his school mates I mean, we might have been able to help him... we were too young you see, too young to understand. When he died, it was just glossed over. None of us knew for sure what had happened to him. There were rumours, but... well we never really grieved him really, but that doesn't mean it didn't affect us. It just made us feel strange and uncomfortable really, because none of us understood, and you know what rumours are like; far worse than the real thing.[4]

This extract outlines further important themes. First, there is the way that adults and children alike tended to underestimate the extent of

3 Atkinson also notes that coroners are more likely to scrutinise the evidence very carefully if it appears that a child may have committed suicide, because it is so hard within our culture for a child to be considered capable of this act.

4 32-year-old male participant.

the boy's unhappiness. From the account, the warning signs were there. The isolation of the boy, for example, his inability to make friends, the notes he had left in his desk. Secondly, the participant points out that he and his peers were unable to understand the boy and that they had difficulty knowing how to begin doing so. This draws attention to the importance of discussing issues, such as relationships, emotions and the effects of behaviour with young people, for example, reference is made to the fact that the boy may have been bullied. Again, the participant recalls that no clear explanations had been given about what had happened. This, as the participant observes, made it difficult for him and his peers to grieve the death of the boy. There is no mention of the funeral. So we can perhaps infer that neither the participant nor his peers attended. These are sensitive issues. Establishing clear-cut solutions and guidelines about how to address them is not easy. There are wider issues to consider. For example, the stigma of suicide and the need for the parents of the dead boy to have some privacy in their grief. Each of the extracts above suggest a strong resistance to the acknowledgement that a young child would be capable of committing suicide. It seems unlikely that we will come up with any definitive answers to this question on the basis of the limited research completed for this book. We can however, explore the question from a variety of perspectives. If we argue that in order to approximate towards any action, we need to understand the meaning assigned to it, we can begin our analysis on the basis of meaning. The construction of meaning is a collaborative psychological project, as we have noted, involving variables such as perception, cognition, emotional and social development. We begin with the question of children's intellectual understanding of death.

Cognitive development and the concept of death

Research on children's emotional development following WW II led to a parallel growth in pioneering work aimed at exploring their understanding of death and dying (Nagy, 1959; Kastenbaum, 1967; Riochlin, 1967). Much of this work has adopted the theoretical framework developed by Piaget (1965) in order to describe children's cognitive development. These studies consistently illustrate that children's understanding of death does not develop in a random or haphazard way, but rather as a general sequence that parallels the broader characteristics he outlined (Jenkins and Cavanaugh, 1985; Kenny, 1998b). Briefly, Piaget observed that children's understanding of the world differed qualitatively from that of adults. They can have difficulties understanding distinctions between different states of being, of consciousness, of 'alive' and 'dead', and between that which is animate and inanimate (Anthony, 1971). In order to understand death, children need the ability to comprehend concepts, such as finality, irreversibility and time. They need to understand that, although cyclical patterns exist in the world, these are not universal. Inability to grasp this explains why so many young children believe that 'after a person has been dead for a while, they will be all right and will get up again' (Kastenbuam, 1981). The development of language is significant. Children cannot always grasp concepts until they have a symbolic means to represent them. Conversely, they have problems conveying what they feel, what they do understand. Language provides the symbols by which meanings are conveyed (Hemmings, 1995; Kenny, 1998b). Death is far too abstract a concept for young children, let alone babies to understand. But, as we discussed in the last section, young infants do have anxieties and fears about separation and abandonment. From the age of around two years, a child may have experienced bereavement, or heard death referred to, but find great difficulty in realising that the deceased will not be coming back. Anthony (*op cit*) observed that young children often imagine death as a 'thing' that is done to people; many will describe a deceased person as having been 'killed'. If death is a 'thing' that can be done to others, it can be assumed that a child might infer that it is a 'thing' that a person can do to oneself. A participant recalls when he was younger that:

> I do remember when I was quite young, I can't remember just how young I was mind, that I would sometimes shout at my parents, or anyone who got up my nose come to think of it, 'I'll kill myself'. I can remember saying that a couple of times, but it never went any further. To be honest, it was a way of letting people know how angry I was, but I never really went any further than that, just coming out with it. Or I'd say, 'I wish I was dead' but again, it was a way of letting people know that I wasn't very happy... I never let my thoughts go any further... it was just a statement, as I recall. But then, I can say that, although my parents never let me have all my own way, if they could see when I said that that I really was unhappy. Then they'd give me a hug, or try to put an end to whatever it was that we were arguing about. They just had this ability, most of

> the time that is, to be firm with me and at the same time let me see that they did love me... like, sometimes my mum would look upset and say something like, 'don't say that. You know that we love you and that we'd be very upset if anything happened to you'.[5]

By the time children reach school age, they understand that death happens to everyone and that it is final. But they still have difficulty thinking of death as the end of existence and as we have noted, they may imagine that the dead exist in a separate dimension. From this perspective, death is considered more a different state of being, than one of non-being. This point comes across quite clearly in the following transcript extract:

> I can remember when I was younger, that, if my mum and dad told me off, or if they didn't give me what I wanted, I'd think to myself 'just wait, you'll be sorry if I die'. Then I'd get a certain amount of comfort from thinking about how sorry they'd be. I sort of, had this idea of looking down on them from heaven or whatever, and feeling very self-righteous about how sorry they would all be. I was quite a bit older when it occurred to me that, if I died, then I wouldn't have the satisfaction of kind of, gloating like that. Because if I died, I'd be dead, I'd not be around to enjoy everyone feeling sorry because they'd upset me.

Understanding of death is concrete rather than abstract. In relation to suicide, the nature of this kind of understanding is quite worrying. If children consider death as another kind of existence, one in which they can look on and observe the living, then some children, if very unhappy, might be motivated to express their unhappiness by attempting suicide. They might possibly succeed. Considering such issues, one becomes mindful of Montessori's (1917) strong disapproval of anything that encourages children to engage in fantasy.[6] Further to this Gorer's (1965) observation that parents sometimes appear to promote concrete thinking in the stories that they tell children about death. A substantial number of studies show that pre-school children have immature concepts of death, understanding it as a temporary restriction, sleep or departure and 'that the dead can be brought back to life spontaneously by administering food, medical treatment or magic' (Wass, 1995). It seems that the ability to consider death as a state of non-being, as nothing, is difficult in adults as well as

5 Male participant aged 25 years.

6 The relevance of Montessori's work in relation to suicide and suicide prevention is further discussed in *Chapter 3*.

children. Kastenbaum (1981) notes that 'this approach to the definition of death has some obvious disadvantages. Most of us are accustomed to thinking of death as something'. We know nothing of nothing, so that when we try to conceive of death in this way 'our minds do not know what to do with themselves unless there is at least a little something to work with'. How do we find suitable solutions to help children resolve their difficulties, when we have, to a large degree, failed to resolve them ourselves?

Although Piaget considered that the stages of cognitive development he outlined were genetically determined, he emphasised the importance of experience and interaction with the environment to facilitate the child's progression through them. Many studies have shown that the turning point in children's understanding of death, comes with their first experience of a bereavement (Kenny, 1998b). It seems from the extract below that experience of bereavement may also help the child to understand the impact that suicide can have on others:

> I can't say that I have ever really thought about suicide, but I do remember that my mum [who had been a nurse] did talk about death and did try to explain things to me. I was quite young when I attended my first funeral, and as well as helping me understand death, it also taught me how upset people were when they lost someone that they loved. I suppose, getting to see how upset people were, did make me realise in a way, that it would be selfish to do something like that. And I mean, I know people say that its not their fault [those who commit suicide] but all the same, I do think that it is a selfish thing to do. I mean, if death is awful, I'm sure it must be a lot worse for people if the person committed suicide. Maybe they don't think about it, maybe that is the kind of thing that people should be talking about, you know, the awful... well terrible really, effect that suicide will have on other people.[7]

Leenaars (1995) argues that suicide is not a moral issue. But it could be argued that there is an inescapable moral aspect to it due to its impact on survivors. It seems from the account given on *page 8* that children may see suicide as a kind of 'divine retribution' a punishment on those who have hurt or betrayed them. Piaget (1932) had observed that young children's perception of moral rules was that these were inflexible and God given. A child who feels betrayed or angered by a parent may be tempted to consider suicide a suitable

7 20-year-old male.

'just world' punishment completed in order to bring home perceived injustices. This is worrying, particularly given the child's rather concrete understanding of death. However, young children's moral orientation could perhaps be facilitated in more positive ways. Drawing on the work of Piaget and Kohlberg some very useful work has been done aimed at facilitating the development of moral reasoning in children (Hersh *et al*, 1980). This approach has a great deal of potential when extended to suicide prevention and mental health promotion. Other participants in this study, who had considered suicide at some time in their lives, said that witnessing the impact that a suicide had on survivors, acted as a deterrent. The participant cited below admitted having made frequent suicide attempts when he was in his 'teens' (the participant did not state at what age these attempts began or stopped). When asked what made him stop making such attempts, he replied:

> What did it for me was, a friend of mine actually did commit suicide. He was about the same age as me, and it was terrible, absolutely terrible the effect that it had on his family, especially his dad. Em... this lad, he'd always been that little bit inclined to get depressed, but his dad did everything for him... it's as if he was afraid, as if he knew that... well you don't know do you? But anyway, when his son died, well the father just went completely to pieces, he really did. And he would not accept, he absolutely would not, that his son had meant to do it... I suppose, when I saw that, and I mean, I have a young family now, and no way would I want to do that to them, to have them grieve like that... so yes, I get down now, but I never, I've not thought about suicide for quite a while... touch wood. Seriously though, once I started thinking about what it would do to other people, I stopped thinking about suicide.[8]

It would be impossible to make generalisations on the basis of the one case cited above. The above account suggests some value in exploring children's moral as well as their cognitive development, in relation to suicide. Indeed, the 'moral dilemmas' approach developed by Kohlberg (1970) may offer some interesting possibilities here.[9] A more complex, abstract understanding of death usually occurs by the

8 32-year-old male participant.

9 The method developed by Kohlberg involves presenting children with a story or moral dilemma that they are encouraged to discuss. One of the dilemmas developed by Kohlberg ('Hans stole the drug') actually does introduce some of the moral issues related to death and dying. It is the view of the author that it would take very little effort to develop similar stories to explore with children the issues of suicide.

time young people reach adolescence, by which time many appear to want to deny it, postpone thinking about it, or, conversely, flirt with it (Wass, 1995). However, some adolescents do attempt and complete suicide attempts (see *Chapter 2*). It appears from our discussion in this chapter that despite any differences in children's understanding of death, they would, if sufficiently distressed, contemplate suicide although the meaning behind the intention to do so would differ from that of adults.

Emotional development

The need to escape from emotional pain may provide a child with the motivation to commit suicide. There is an abundance of historical, clinical and case study evidence to suggest that children do experience despair, hopelessness and depression, and that this can lead to suicidal thoughts. Research, conducted at the University of Queensland (1998), concluded that younger children are at greater risk precisely because of the lower rate of completed suicide in this age group. As with the case cited above, the rarity of the phenomenon can lead to complacency. The researchers also inferred that lower suicide completions in younger children may indicate less opportunity rather than lower intent. Young children are more likely to be supervised. They are likely to have restricted access to suicide aids, such as tablets or guns. The researchers observed that hanging is one of the most common methods used by children who commit suicide (most houses have ropes and these are rarely supervised).[10] So the availability of aids required to complete an act of suicide is important, as too is the intellectual ability to plan it successfully.

Children are disadvantaged in both respects, but this does not mean that they lack the motive if sufficiently distressed. The researchers caution against assumptions that we may be less concerned about child suicide. They note that depression and despair are also less likely to be identified in young children who are less able to express their feelings in words and less inclined to talk about their problems. This makes suicide risk in younger children harder to identify, predict and prevent. For those who experience a bereavement due to a suicide, it can be this unpredictability that makes the grieving process so

10 It is on the basis of such evidence that Mercy (1997) argues that restricting access to lethal means is an important step in suicide prevention. Older adolescents on the other hand, use a variety of methods, including guns, drugs or other substances.

difficult. At what age might a child contemplate or attempt suicide due to emotional trauma? At a very young age it seems. Frommer (1968) observed depressive symptoms in children as young as four years of age. Symptoms included 'difficulty in getting off to sleep, restlessness, nightmares, sleepwalking, talking or screaming and early morning waking'.[11] Frommer also observed that a significant number of suicidal children made quite clear and explicit statements about their depressive feelings. A minority had difficulty expressing such feelings verbally and presented instead with indirect expressions of distress. Symptoms included: loss of appetite, tummy pains, headaches or psychological features, such as boredom, fatigue and lack of concentration. Depressed children are also reported to make statements such as 'I wish I were dead' or 'you'll be sorry if I die'. Of course, many children say things such as this if they feel unhappy or angry with their families or peers. However, they should be taken seriously if they are made repeatedly.

Some of the earliest systematic studies of maternal deprivation were conducted during and just after World War II (Dominian, 1990). These studies observed the emotional reactions of children who had been separated from their parents for a variety of reasons and placed in institutions. Although very systematic and thorough, there was a tendency in all this research to look for the one commonality these children shared (that is, absence of the mother) and to exclude all others (eg. overcrowding, lack of intellectual stimulation, absence of a father). We noted in the introduction, value assumptions (ie. 'where are you coming from?') form the basis for all thought, all questions and enquiry. If you believe that the mother is the only suitable person to bring up children, then it is understandable that this is the one variable that you will focus on. This is not to suggest that the findings of such studies were invalid. It does suggest however that their conclusions offered insights that were partial and biased.

Dominian (*op cit*) cites a study conducted in 1946 by Spitz and Wolf, in which the reactions of children separated from their imprisoned mothers were observed. Reactions reported included, 'misery, lack of expression and withdrawal'.[12] These findings correspond with those made by Burlington and Freud (1944) who had observed a group of children who had survived the concentration camps. Unlike the children in the Spitz and Wolfe sample, this

11 This is also common in adult sufferers of endogenous depression.
12 These were later described by Spitz as 'anaclitic' depressions.

second group had learned to draw on each other for support, but they had done this at the expense of becoming 'inwardly' focused, and were very suspicious of any 'outsiders'. Work by John Bowlby (1979) and his co worker, Mary Ainsworth, added further importance to the process of parent/child bonding and attachment, and also to the effects of separation, which included intense grieving and a sequence of protest, despair and detachment (Bowlby, *op cit*; Ainsworth and Wittig, 1969).

For young children and babies it is separation that causes distress. They have no conceptual understanding of death *per se* (Dyregrow and Kingsley, 1991). Repeated, insecure separations (where no familiar substitute is provided) can lead to a process described by Klein (1960) as 'splitting' — the repression of painful memories that are assigned to the unconscious. This can lead to a depletion in the ego and a resultant 'fragmentation' of the personality that, if extreme, poses serious threats to mental health in later life (Brown and Harris, 1978; Douglas, 1989). Psychologists, such as Piaget and Bruner (cited by Bee, 1985), have shown that children lack the required cognitive competence to build up detailed declarative memories (Van r Kolk *et al*, 1984; Squire, 1994).[13] Early and/or traumatic memories are often sensual rather than conceptual in nature. However, sensory memories based on early trauma can lead to the occurrence of 'flashbulb' memories in adulthood (Brown and Kulik, 1977; Briere and Conte, 1993). This can lead to conditions, such as agoraphobia (fear of open spaces) that appear irrational, but can be distressing enough to drive a person to suicide. They can also lead to the formulation of a very negative self-concept, which is internalised in such a way that the person considers themselves to be in a state of putrefaction (Crook, 1992). Repressed memories can also lead to a form of emotional detachment that Lifton (1973) refers to as 'emotional deadness'. This is a fear of displaying emotions in case self-control is lost completely (Shaton, 1973). This frequently contributes to suicidal feelings (sometimes apparently irrational), risk behaviours and substance abuse in later life (Bluementhal and Kupfer, 1990; Goodwin, 1987). A young child's limited linguistic skills can make it difficult to convey feelings, although these can be expressed by other forms, such as through nursery rhymes (Higgins, 1993). Choice of inappropriate words, from an adult point of view, can also lead to misunderstandings and conflict (Lendrum and Syme, 1992).

13 Declarative memory refers to a conscious awareness of facts or events that have happened to the individual.

In 1972, Balkwin (who was then Professor of Clinical Pediatrics in New York) observed that, in the first half of this century, death rates for institutionalised infants had been nearly 100%.[14] Many of these children failed to thrive, even when eating an adequate diet.[15] Further investigation revealed this to be a widespread phenomenon also reported in Europe, Latin America as well as the USA. This lethargy, lack of interest in life and apparent lack of a will to live could be considered a form of suicidal intent in very young children. If such children were removed from the institutional context and placed with a substitute mothering figure, the change was dramatic and striking. Balkwin attributed this 'marasmus' to lack of exposure to sensory stimulation, and to lack of contact with a mother or nurse. Deprivation studies have been invaluable in drawing our attention to the emotional needs of the child. But children from apparently secure homes can also be very unhappy and, indeed, at times suicidal. It seems that even in the absence of neglect or abuse, communication can break down between parents and children. A child is just as capable of misinterpreting other people's behaviour (including that of his/her parents) as anyone else. Relationships can disintegrate if children receive the wrong messages. This causes distress that may be expressed in behavioural problems, such as temper tantrums, separation fears and sleeping difficulties (Talley, 1998).

Dominian (*op cit*) describes such a breakdown in the parent/child relationship. He cites the case of a young American boy who began making suicide attempts at the age of three and a half years of age.[16] The boy was the eldest in a family of three children. His mother had a difficult pregnancy, so there may have been some difficulties in the attachment formation process.[17] By the time he was five months old, the boy was having quite severe temper tantrums. Even at this early age, Dominian attributed the child with characteristics, such as bossiness, aggression and negativity. However, Dominian also observed characteristics, such as talkability and over activity in his character assessment, attributes that could indicate a

14 This study is cited by Dominian, 1990.

15 Balkwin called this condition 'Hospitalismus'.

16 This child's first suicide attempt happened when he threw himself out of a first storey window.

17 Dominian describes this particular mother as 'intellectually dull', but he makes no attempt to clearly define what he means by this. In the absence of further evidence, we should not exclude the fact that Dominian may have been observing some mild depression in the mother and/or perhaps cultural or class differences in behavioural conduct that he was unable to understand.

high level of intelligence for a child of this age. The boy did not 'fit in' at home or at school. By the time he was four years old, he was making suicide threats whenever his misbehaviour was checked or punished. The parents responded as positively as they could. But they must have experienced a great deal of stress and this may have been conveyed unintentionally to their son. Dominian provides no follow-up information on how the boy fared as a young adult, or of whether he ever actually managed to complete a suicide attempt, but this case study is useful in that it shows how suicidal behaviour is often due to several factors. Clearly, there are other psychological issues that we need to take into account, such as the role of social learning.

Social learning approaches

The family provides the first basic, primary social unit of the child's interactive, social world. As such, it provides a basis for learning basic human skills and attitudes and beliefs. Social learning theory emphasises the importance of the environment and of role models (Bandura, 1977). If a child is reared in an environment where his or her adult role models regularly express violent, aggressive or pessimistic outlooks, then there is a strong possibility that the child will develop similar attitudes to life. Research suggests that suicides are more common in children and young people who come from 'dysfunctional' families (Samaritans, 1998). However, we must also be sensitive to the fact that social problems outside a family's control can be the cause of such 'dysfunctions'. A family history of mental health problems, substance abuse and family violence, which includes physical or sexual abuse, can place a young person at greater risk of committing suicide. Depressed children who have such family backgrounds are more likely to be suicidal then depressed young people who come from 'stable' families. Parents, who are very ambitious and keen to establish middle-class lifestyles, may be under a great deal of stress and, as a result, 'hurry' their children (Elkind, 1981). Families provide role models for young people. Exposure to the suicidal behaviour of others, including family members, peers, or even important media role models, increases risk. The presence of such role models can lead the child to consider that suicidal behaviour is an acceptable means to draw attention to his or her distress.

The family environment can greatly increase the risk of suicide, for example, children and young people's exposure or accessibility to suicide aids. The United States of America 1995 suicide statistics revealed that use of fire arms accounted for 59% of suicides in men and women. Some families have a very low tolerance to any kind of crisis and respond aggressively. Aggressive ways of managing crisis often have historical links. These are likely to be hard to break, given that they have probably developed over several generations. In such a context, the suicide is not so much a passive victim, but rather a participator in a communication process in which conflict is typically handled by aggressive means. In the case of suicide, this aggression is directed at the self, but it communicates something. The same argument can be related to self-mutilation whether or not the act constitutes direct harm, or a suicide attempt. The message conveyed goes something like this, 'see how you are cutting me up' (Aldridge, 1998).

The family is not the only source of role models. Popular culture provides many powerful role models, and these can have a profound impact on young people's perceptions and behaviour. They may be relatively rare, but there are accounts of spates of 'copycat' suicide epidemics. Leenaar (1995) observes that, historically, there have been times when suicide has been romanticised and even quite fashionable. He cites the case of the publication of Johann Wolfgang von Goethe's book (1749–1832) *The Sorrows of Young Werther*. Following rejection by his lover, the main character of the book, young Werther, kills himself. The book had quite an impact on the young of the time. The clothes that young Werther had worn became fashionable; so too, became the act of suicide in response to unrequited love. Other 'copycat' effects have been recorded. In the 1970s, an 18-year-old Japanese pop idol, Yikko Okada, committed suicide after an argument with her lover. In the first 17 days following her death, 33 young people, all Yikko Okada fans, committed suicide. Suicide can also be associated with glamour and success, for example, in the cases of people such as Monroe and Janis Joplin (Wertheimer, 1991) and in the rhythm and lyrics of violent rock music (Wass *et al*, 1989). Television is perhaps the most common media through which role models are exposed. It is not clear, however, to what extent this might influence suicidal behaviour (Wass, 1995). Younger people, especially adolescents, appear to be particularly vulnerable to violent media representations (Stack, 1991), although some of the young people who took part in Kenny's study (1998c) challenged this assumption.

We need to consider the positive impact that social learning can have on young people. Crook (1992) has stressed the importance of the parental role in a study of teenage suicidal behaviour. The study emphasised the importance of the need for parents to listen to their children rather than lecturing them, and of helping children cope with stress and emotional pain. Crook also observed the importance of parents teaching independence to their children, while remaining involved and supportive, and of helping to build the child's self-confidence and self-esteem. Rioch (1994) also asserts the importance of discussing emotional and mental health problems with young people, openly and in supportive environments, such as the home, classroom and school clinic. This may help to remove the stigma associated with such issues, and of course, if we relate this to our present discussion, parents and others present excellent role models if they do this in a calm, non-threatening manner that suggests these matters are open to discussion. Indeed, if we are to accept the basic principles of social learning theory, then children learn best from the behaviour of the role models to which they are exposed. If the child is raised in an environment where available role models are observed to be emotionally strong, flexible individuals with a range of coping strategies, it is likely that he or she will develop similar coping strategies. In the next section we consider challenge, crisis and how people's responses to these change over the lifespan.

Lifespan developmental approaches

Many of the theoretical approaches that we have discussed so far focus on early child development. Erikson was one of the first theorists to develop an analysis of psychological change and development throughout the lifespan. He did this by extending Freud's psychoanalytical approach to include a further three stages, each conceptualised as an interactive process. This involved a process of establishing compromise between the child's needs, the maturing ego and the social world. A strong theme that remains consistent throughout is that of **trust**, a theme that, as we have already discussed, appears to be increasingly problematic in post-modernity. 'Greed is probably one of the first emotions experienced by the young child. Children hungrily take in all the things that they need, and more, but must also learn that these demands cannot always be met immediately' (Benedek, 1938). Frustration is best tolerated if the child has confidence in the consistency and reliability of their caretakers. Parents differ in the way that they deliver care. They may attend promptly to the child's needs, or they may follow a strict regime. To establish trust, it is not so much the method that matters, as the level of consistency demonstrated. Once trust in others is established, trust in self follows. 'A very young baby, for example, may nip the breast and the mother (naturally) responds to this. If her response is firm but not violent, the child learns (without intimidation) that this is not an appropriate way to behave. The child learns to trust him/herself not to lose control' (Crain, 1980). The ability to trust self and others is an important starting point in the development of self-efficacy skills in later life (Bandura *et al*, 1961). Trust is also essential if the child is to develop independence, confidence and the ability to cope with separation.[18] Bradshaw (1965) found that children are very resilient and have an 'innate optimism and trust in people'. He argues that children's perceptions generally operate on the assumption that the world is a friendly place. However, trust and optimism can be blunted through misunderstanding, insecurity or violation from a parent, or other source.

Erikson was concerned about the importance of confidence in parents. If the child is to develop trust in the parent, then the parents must have confidence in themselves. He noted that inconsistent advice given by child experts could undermine the confidence of parents. This is why Erikson emphasised that it was not so much method that matters, but rather consistency.[19] When children reach the ages of two to three years, conflict can emerge due to the struggle to achieve some independence. A child wants to develop in the way that his or her inclinations demand, while the parent has a responsibility to teach the child the socially acceptable way to behave. This is a delicate stage and it can be very difficult to strike a balance. If balance is not achieved, shame and doubt might develop instead of independence. Doubt develops from the knowledge that one is not so powerful after all. To a point this is helpful. It is, after all, realistic. The child has to learn to accommodate the feelings of others. Parents best enable the child to develop autonomy by allowing them gradual independence.

18 Children also need to develop mistrust, otherwise they are unable to distinguish when trust is appropriate and when it is not. It is not so much the development of trust or mistrust that is important, but rather that the child develops a favourable balance between the two, and that basic trust should predominate. Erikson (1976) stated that 'it is clear that the human infant must experience a goodly share of mistrust in order to trust wisely'.

19 Erikson was also a great advocate of the work of Spock, because the latter believed that parents should have the confidence to be guided by their intuitive knowledge of the child.

The next stage of crisis to emerge is that of initiative versus guilt. By now the child has realised that 'their biggest plans and fondest hopes are doomed to failure'. In Freudian terms, a superego, or conscience emerges (Crain, 1980). The child internalises social prohibitions. The superego is necessary for social life, but it initiates a crisis because of its potential to stifle initiative. By the time the child has reached six to seven years of age, they have usually learned to channel their ambitions into realistic, attainable and socially acceptable goals. The period between ages six and seven are, from Erikson's perspective very creative, but potentially traumatic. This stage involves development of more advanced aspects of ego expansion as the child shifts towards adulthood and all the responsibilities this shift entails.[20] 'Acutely aware of the new responsibilities, the child struggles to master important cognitive and social skills' (Crain, 1980). Erikson referred to this as a period of industry versus inferiority. Children go to school, socialise more openly and are asked to master skills, such as reading, writing and arithmetic. Failure can be the source of strong feelings of inferiority and relate to social as well as scholastic skills. Children who fail at school may not 'fit in', although much depends on the social value placed on education within any particular subgroup. Alternatively, a child may do very well at school, but learn that due, for example, to their social class or the colour of their skin, no amount of scholarly success is noticed or indeed matters in relation to how much they are socially accepted. This too, of course, can lead to feelings of inferiority rather than industry. From the case study presented at the start of this chapter (*p. 8*), we noted that an inability to fit in can have quite serious psychological consequences.

In this last section we introduce the reader to the first, childhood stage of Erikson's theory of lifespan development. We have discussed how the development of trust and confidence in the reliability of caregivers contributes to the development of self-efficacy skills, and the ability to develop independence. Independence is an important requirement if the child is to enjoy and fully benefit from the creative learning potential offered by the early school years. It is also important if the young person, having reached adolescence, is to deal successfully with separation. For the purpose of this research, the main strength of Erikson's theory, is that the terminology he used to describe the stages he identified (eg. trust, intimacy, despair)

20 Freud had referred to this as the latency period. In contrast to Erikson, Freud considered this to be a time of relative calm compared to the conflict associated with the earlier stages.

reflected universal human experience.[21] As such, many people can relate to them. In the next chapter we explore Erikson's theory further in relation to adolescence and early adulthood development.

Conclusion

Taken collectively, the psychological approaches discussed in this chapter support the assumption that depression and suicidal thoughts can be present in very young children. However, given that children's intellectual understanding of death is very different from that of adults, we need to acknowledge that for a child the meaning behind a suicide attempt may be very different. We noted that it is precisely children's immature understanding of death that may place them at greater risk, and that this potential risk might be underestimated due to the lower rates of completed suicide in the young.[22] Children and young people may attempt suicide for a variety of reasons. They may feel unsure of their own worth, a feeling that may be excessive due to early experiences of rejection. Young people may have problems establishing and/or maintaining relationships. They may have social skills that, within a particular context, are inappropriate or appear inadequate. They may perceive that the relationships that they have are not as satisfactory as they would like them to be. Such perceptions stem from a variety of sources. A personal history of frustrated, unsatisfied attachment needs may lead to mistrust, lack of confidence and insecure, demanding approaches to relationships. Attempts to address such a complex issue as child suicide need to be very diverse and flexible.

21 We develop this discussion further in *Chapter 3*.
22 Biological factors also play a part, although these are not discussed in this book.

2

Adolescence and early adulthood

Introduction

It is common to associate the start of adolescence with puberty and its termination with early adulthood.[1] Dominian considers the average age of marriage as the turning point of adolescence to early adulthood. Adolescence is also commonly associated with 'storm and strife', a view challenged by Bandura (1980). It can be difficult to distinguish between the characteristics of 'normal' and (unfortunately) painful processes of growing up and those that indicate the development of depression and possible suicidal thoughts. Adolescence can be a confused period, with blurred and sometimes contradictory rites of passage. A young person of 16 years cannot vote, but he or she can marry (Hollinger, 1978; Pasho, 1998; Royal College of Psycholgists, 1998b). Changes in patterns of labour have led to an expansion in further and higher education. The age at which young people can expect to live an independent life now extends into the period once associated with early adulthood (Holland, 1975). Despite its ambiguity, adolescence is also quite a positive stage in the lifespan. Adolescents have a more sophisticated understanding of death and because of this, a greater motivation to assign some meaning and purpose to their lives (Becker, 1991). They have sufficient mastery of language to express their thoughts and feelings. Their ability to engage in abstract thinking opens up new and exciting possibilities for self-definition and growth.

According to Erikson, adolescence and early adulthood signify a gradual progression through the stages of identity (*v.* role confusion), intimacy (*v.* isolation and self-absorption) and finally, generativety. The stage that signifies early adulthood, generativety, is symbolic of the acquired psychological maturity required to make long-term commitments. Successful transition through these stages depends upon issues, such as the support systems available, the coping skills of the young individual and on the earlier establishment

1 At the time that Dominion wrote this, in 1990, this was around age 24 years for men and 22 years for women.

of trust. Erikson believed that young people require a period of psycho-social moratorium, that is, 'time out' to find themselves. In Erikson's youth it was common for the 'better off' young to do this. Erikson did this himself as did many other psychologists, such as Jung and Piaget, before they made a commitment to a career (Crain, 1980). The opportunities that your social class make available to you are clearly very important. Young working-class people have rarely had such opportunities. At the present time, politicians and moralists consider the young unemployed to be 'wasters' and there is no assumption that they might be on some kind of 'spiritual journey'. However, regardless of whether or not young people have such socially sanctioned periods of 'time out', they frequently progress through a 'drifting phase'. They may experience a consequent lack of any real sense of identity because of their inability to commit to anything. This can lead to depression and, if severe, suicide.

If young people make commitments too soon, ie. in relation to their own psycho-social development, they risk 'identity fore-closure'. This is a premature commitment to compartmentalised, externally assigned social roles for which they are ill fitted. If they have children, for example, they risk neglecting the children's emotional needs.[2] The ability to self-reflect is an important part of positive self-development and is, by necessity, self-interested.[3] Failure to develop generativity may be due to an impoverished childhood. There may be a lack of opportunity to 'find' one's self. Western culture values self-fulfilment and personal achievement. This can discourage concern for others. The following sections discuss progression through the stages of adolescence to early adulthood, examining some of the crisis and conflicts that can lead to depression and suicide in young people.

2 However, it is here that the theory has an implicit sexism. For, in practice, it is women rather than men (as a general rule) who are expected to demonstrate their maturity by putting needs and ambitions of others before their own. Men, on the other hand, traditionally spend much of their working lives prioritising their creative 'needs' in pursuit of a career. For them, this is not neglect of responsibility, but rather acceptance of it.

3 The author accepts that self-reflection can become excessive, introspective and counterproductive. Nevertheless, she considers self-reflection to be important because it is of little use having any commitment to any principles, if one is unable to explore one's own assumptions and prejudice. It is amazing that many people support 'just' causes, but can go through life entirely unaware of their own prejudices and biases. The behavioural principle, 'do as I say, not as I do' comes about less through arrogance and more from a belief that others are ignorant while the self is enlightened.

Detachment, separation and identity

Within Erikson's framework, identity versus role confusion is one of the earliest causes of conflict to emerge during adolescence. The detachment theme provides one of the most potent catalysts at this stage. Families have become more fragmented, diverse, open and unstable, at least in traditional terms. Transitions symbolic to adulthood, such as marriage and employment can demand that younger members move, sometimes many miles away from their roots. Education and employment may also lead to the young adult changing from one social class to another. Aldridge (1998) suggests that transition to adulthood also involves disengagement. Some families (and indeed, the young person's subgroup) may interpret attempts to disengage as disloyal. 'The most dramatic changes in all organisations occur when someone enters or leaves' (Aldridge, *op cit*). In some families the parents may have drifted apart, so that the child (or children) is the only remaining interest that they share. Undue pressure may be put on the child to stay. This may stabilise the family temporarily, but crisis will be inevitable if the young person has no real desire to stay.

Ironically, the position may be more problematic if the parents feel ambivalent about the child staying. They are aware that, generally in Western society, it may be considered pathological for an adult child to stay with his or her parents forever, but, at the same time, they fear separation. The young person receives mixed and confusing messages — go! stay! In circumstances such as these, the young person may be driven to attempt suicide. The unconscious motivation may be that this might bring about some stability. It is common, in the event of a crisis, for families to forget their differences and all attention is diverted to the suicidal person. Aldridge (*op cit*) emphasises an interactive process whereby:

> *A suicidal attempt has been seen as a bid by one member of a social group to communicate his distress to those intimately associated with him and that the attempt functions as part of a language. If suicidal behaviour is part of a language, it is not an individual phenomenon but a social phenomenon.*

Aldridge further notes that:

> *Such a view emphasises that suicidal behaviour by one member is part of a social process and is not an initiator of a sequence of behaviour nor is it the result of being a passive*

> *victim. In other words, the suicidal member of a social group does not communicate but participates in communication.*

To paraphrase Aldridge further, some family theorists argue on this basis that suicidal behaviour exhibited by young people in some cases may be 'benevolent' (if misguided) rather than 'deviant'. It is a reflection of the young person's attempt to stabilise conflict. In times of crisis, most families begin to 'pull together'. From this perspective, suicide attempts in such situations become a stabilising device that maintains survival of family unity. This scenario more frequently occurs when parents and child have a very strong 'symbolic attachment' to each other. This tolerates no measure of autonomy on the part of any individual. Detachment in such circumstances involves tension between maintaining some coherence within the family while, at the same time, seeking independence outside. What distinguishes such families from those in which a strong but healthy attachment exists? In such cases, the parent is more emotionally dependent on the child than vice versa. Such parents may persistently interfere and insist on being informed about all aspects of the child's life. Yet they withdraw if unable to provide support when it is needed. Typically, such parents deny their children any opportunity to be children. They insist that the child acts like a miniature adult at all times, but deny them all the opportunities required to develop the independence of thought that is an integral part of adulthood.[4] The threat of death by suicide in such a context, may reflect underlying family conflict brought about by the threat of change (Aldridge, *op cit*). Tragically, there are times when attempted suicides are completed; the young person dies.

Gould (1978) considered that separation to achieve psychological status as an adult requires a 'letting go' of the assumption that 'I am theirs' to the recognition that 'I own myself'. Belonging to 'them' is comforting. It provides security. The prospect of separation can seem awesome to young people. They may be shy, timid and afraid of leaving the protection of the family. They may have great difficulty admitting (even to themselves) that there is a problem because, 'youth is a time when there can be no fear, its admission can be intensely humiliating' (Dominian, 1990). To a point, such difficulties are not surprising when we consider what separation means for the young adult. As part of the separation process, young

4 In other words, the child is an adult until whatever time it suits the parent to allocate them back to childhood status, an action which is often asserted to disempower the child and re-assert parental control.

people have to strike a balance between the need to be true to themselves without, at the same time, jeopardising long-term relationships. This can all seem very threatening. The ability to cope with life crisis and trauma is an important 'buffer' against suicide. Young people have little experience, and may have relatively low apprehension of their self-efficacy skills (Rotter *et al*, 1972; Bandura, 1982). They may consider themselves unable to adjust to change, especially that initiated by crisis (Adler, 1910/1967, cited by Wass, 1995). The person's psychological state may be incompatible with the changes required. He/she may consider him/herself inadequate, unable to cope. As people age, they learn from practical experience that they are able to cope. Ironically, this ability can grow from experiencing and surviving the kinds of traumas that have been the cause of suicidal thoughts when the person was younger. A female participant in her forties (who admitted to having had suicidal thoughts when she was younger) made the following comments:

> I think that it is very sad, but all the same I think that younger people do run a more serious risk of suicide, especially adolescents, because in one way they are mature, and in another they are not. What I mean is, they are just starting to meet up with stress, and responsibility and love... well young people have this romantic idea of everlasting love. So if their girlfriend or boyfriend finishes with them, they can really believe that it is the end of the world. Whereas, the older you get, the more experience you get of stress and of broken relationships. And you get to realise that you survive, that you can build your life again, love again and all this. In a way it can be handy to have some stress in your life because the more you have to cope with it the more confident you get that you can cope with it. It makes you stronger in some ways. I mean, I've been through all sorts. I've had some really, really hard and stressful times. And yes, there really have been times when I felt that I really could have 'topped' myself. But the good thing about that is that I've reached a time in my life when I can look back and think 'well, I coped with this and I coped with that, so I can cope with anything'. You see, the more experiences of dealing with stress and so forth that you get, the more stress changes, that is, the way that you see it. So when you've had a lot of stress and survived, you get sort of immune to it. I don't mean that you don't feel it. Of course you do, you wouldn't be human if you didn't. But at the same time, no matter how awful it is, you know it's not forever. Now a younger person hasn't got that experience. I can look back now and remember times when I was young, and the situation

> seemed so awful, life just didn't seem to be worth living at all. And now those times are such a long time ago, and I've had good experiences in between the bad, that I would never have had if I'd have 'topped' myself during the times that I'd felt bad. But now I think, 'thank God I didn't, because if I had, then I wouldn't have had all the good times that I've had, all the good times that I'm going to have — as well as the bad times'. [5]

The participant above has been fortunate. She has managed to survive life's traumas and has, perhaps, become a stronger person because of it. However, she also points out that this has been an agonising process, one that stems from direct, lived experience. It is an outlook to life that reflects a certain level of maturity. This raises questions. The participant admitted to having considered suicide many times. She did not admit to having attempted it. Despite all her traumas, there are some aspects of this woman's life history that protected her, ultimately, from considering suicide a reasonable option. What makes the distinction between those young (or indeed older) people who contemplate suicide, those who attempt, and those who go on to complete? The literature offers limited clues. Many people have negative experiences that place them at risk. Many have insecure family backgrounds, feeling that they do not fit and are alienated, but they do not attempt suicide. If we examine the extract above more closely, there are some helpful themes that may enable the development of coping skills. The first is the ability to reflect, to provide a critical and realistic assessment of one's strengths and weaknesses. There exists an ability to cherish the bad times as well as the good, an ability to make balanced attributions (Abramson *et al*, 1978). This reflects an appreciation that, while personal agency is important, other forces exist outside the individual's control (Wallston and Wallston, 1978). There are many themes in the above extract that suggest that the speaker has acquired the essential skills required for adult development. Such skills include, the ability to shoulder responsibility, to make logical decisions, to cope with minor frustrations and to accept one's social role (Sugerman, 1986).

Shakespeare (1996) argues that 'identity is an aspect of the stories that we tell to ourselves and others'. The value of balanced reflection (or self-storytelling) is that it can culminate in an understanding that all experiences in life, even the bad ones, are worthwhile. All experience provides a valuable basis for learning.

5 A 45-year-old woman who reported that she has often considered suicide but never attempted it.

Such human attributes are unlikely to develop unless the person is fairly confident, self-assured and has a strong sense of who they are. Identity is clearly an integral part of this. As we have noted, all suicides, attempted or completed, signify the climax of a complex biography. Some young people who commit suicide may have appeared to have had everything. Or do they? When the researcher posed this question to one of the funeral directors who took part in this study, he responded 'if you commit suicide love, you've not got everything going for you!'

The biography of Justin Fastanu supports the view expressed above. Justin became a football star at a very early age.[6] In his prime he was proclaimed a 'super-hero', 'sensational' 'awesome' the 'black panther' of soccer. As a successful professional, Justin provided a positive role model for other black youths. Yet despite his success, Justin's life was torn by conflicts of identity. A strong public identity had been assigned to him by virtue of his success. What effect might this have on the private experience of the man? There were many aspects of Justin's personality that conflicted with his public image. According to the BBC documentary on his life, the news that Justin had attended gay clubs, initially brought bad publicity. This was met with some hostility by the black and football community. Both express very traditional notions about men and masculinity. Religion offered a source of comfort and he became a born again Christian. Unhappily, this was not enough to ease the apparent emptiness that he felt inside. Justin eventually committed suicide.

Given Justin's success, his suicide may seem inexplicable. His biography certainly provides a challenge to some of the causes often attributed to youth suicide, such as unemployment and poverty. Justin's struggles appear to have been more closely connected to self-concept, identity, the conflict between his professional self, his sexuality and his struggle to find some sense of belonging. Perhaps Justin was ill equipped to deal with wealth and fame at such a young age. And yet for many young people, limited possibilities for an independent life might contribute towards the development of depression and suicide. In the following discussion we consider some of these themes, and the way that they may contribute to youth unhappiness and, possibly, suicide. We begin with sexuality.

6 BBC1, 'Inside Story of Fallen Hero', Justin Fastanu, Thursday, 3 September 1998.

Sexuality and identity

Whether we consider it in relation to biology, gender or sexual preference, sexuality has become a very significant means of defining ourselves and our identity:

> *Gender and sexuality provide two of the most basic narratives through which our identities are forged. For most people, identity is first of all a gender category, but its characteristics are thought to derive from fundamental differences in male and female sexuality. These differences are often expressed in terms of natural or biological difference. In the West at least, we live in subjective worlds, where the dynamics of gender, tied in with heterosexual imperatives (or our resistance to them) provide the foundations for our sense of self.*
>
> Segal, 1997

Yet at the same time (given that this concept has also been deconstructed, challenged and scrutinised) it has, perhaps, become even more problematic. The post-modernist celebration of difference and diversity has brought costs as well as benefits. What is femininity, masculinity, homosexuality, etc? In challenging taken-for-granted assumptions, definitions and boundaries have become blurred, intangible and invisible. This may have caused insecurities for women and men, especially the young who are struggling to establish their sexual self.

Young people can become very unhappy if they consider themselves unattractive, and this can have fearful consequences for their mental health. Distinctions between masculinity and femininity, and for many, identification with these constructions of identity, also become very significant. Indeed, one participant gave some compelling thoughts on why he considers that more young men complete suicide:[7]

> A friend of mine committed suicide — he threw petrol over himself. And I think that a man is more likely to choose a violent method. Its about being a man you see? A man mustn't fail. Not even, and maybe especially even in something like that. I mean, for a man to be seen as like 'crying for help'. He'd never live it down like, people saying 'oh, he never meant to do

7 This participant was in his mid-thirties. The friend he refers to committed suicide when the two were in their early twenties.

> it', you know? If you are a man then you are going to show that you can do it, it's this macho thing, you mustn't fail. You must prove yourself in everything, even something like that.

The above account suggests that there can be an intense determination to confirm gender identity. It provides a harrowing reminder of what can happen when only violent outlets are available for the expression of powerful emotions.[8] The pervasive assumptions about so called 'natural' differences between the sexes, apparently influences, not just the methods of suicide chosen, but the way that action is interpreted by survivors. A point made clear by the participant cited below:

> One thing that is noticeable in our job is that there are definitely differences in the way that men and women do it [commit suicide]. I mean, a lot of the men who commit suicide that we get in, have done it by violent means, you know, they put their head on a railway track, hang themselves or whatever. Now women, they don't like to make a mess, especially housewives. It really is astonishing how many women cut their wrists in the bath. And they'll take a lot more care about making sure that it's tidy, and that whoever finds them will not have to cope too much with shock and mess and all this. It does make you wonder, doesn't it? [9]

Freud attributed the 'storm' and 'strife' so characteristic of adolescence to the revival of earlier oedipal fantasies (Dominian, 1990). Young people often have immense sexual energy, but they usually direct these feelings to the establishment of relationships, not always with the opposite sex. The young person can place a great emotional investment into these early relationships. He/she may react violently to rejection which may be the 'last straw' leading to suicide. Two of the participants in this study have been involved with a person whose suicide was attributed to unhappy romantic involvement. One participant noted with regret that younger people lack the life experience to recognise the possibility of recovering from romantic disappointments, to love and live again:

> Adults often make the mistake of assuming that children and young people are not as intelligent as them, if you see what I mean, that they don't really understand things like relationships. They [adults] make the mistake of thinking that

8 The author acknowledges that the state of mind of the deceased may well have been influenced by the fact that, according to the storyteller, he had been on drugs. However, Kenny still considers the case representative of some of the extreme emotions that young people can experience.

9 A 42-year-old mortuary employee.

> 'puppy love' as they call it, isn't serious. But when they call it infatuation, to a young person it's not. To that young person, it's real, the pain they feel is real. God! I remember the first girl I really liked who finished with me. I really really felt that the whole world had fallen apart... to be honest, I was too miserable to think of anything, even suicide.[10]

For a young person, possibly far more than for an older person, rejection in love can seem like 'the end of the world'. Lesbians and gay men encounter greater problems, with an increased suicide risk (Bell and Weinberg, 1978). Three working-class, non-academic gay men participated in this study.[11] Their experience of coming out should be interpreted within the context of a specific working-class notion of masculinity, based on toughness, rejection of traditional authorities (including education) and of very clear-cut gender divisions in labour, but not in the way that this might be understood in middle-class terms.[12] Markowe (1997) is sensitive to the social, historical and cultural aspects of 'coming out', making her work an important contribution to the (generally) individualistic orientation of psychology. She cites Hetrick and Martin (1987) who asserted that adjusting to a 'socially stigmatised role' was 'the major task of the gay adolescent'. She further notes that 'the seriousness of problems during adolescence for gay and lesbian young people is reflected in findings of approximately 20% reporting suicide attempts before the age of 20–21 years of age'. However, guilt and stigma can be balanced by feelings of liberation. This ambiguity can, in itself, cause problems. The gay participant cited below recalls his first homosexual encounter:[13]

10 A 43-year-old man remembers the break up of his first romantic relationship. He reported having felt suicidal at various stages in his life, but never going on to attempt it.

11 Although (as Markowe notes) there are important differences between the experience of coming out for men and women.

12 There is insufficient space in this text to discuss these differences, except to note that all three of these young men came from working-class homes where the women had worked full and part-time.

13 Conversations with a 42- and a 45-year-old gay man, and a later conversation with a 23-year-old gay man. It is worth noting here that the younger gay man reported that he had not encountered so many problems 'coming out'. Indeed, he reported that his family and friends supported him. This was unlike the accounts given by the older gay men. None of the gay men interviewed however, would agree to having the conversation taped, although they were happy for me to take notes. This suggests that although attitudes may be more positive than in the past, the very fact that all three of these men were particularly concerned that they should not be identified, suggests some negativism.

> The first time that I did it, I felt physically sick, in fact I was. I just went home and was sick, I thought to myself, 'how could you do that'. But then I thought, 'well you've done it now'. And in a weird sort of way, I felt good about it, I mean, I'd done it, I'd crossed that barrier... and I could do it now, be honest I mean. I mean, no matter what anyone else told me, I knew that for me it was 'normal'. It was like a rebellion in a way, like saying 'up yours' to all of those who had made 'poof' jokes, and made me feel 'abnormal'. I felt good, but I also felt lonely... I mean, back in the 1960s it wasn't as talked about then, not as public. I had a feeling there must be others like me. But how could I find out about them?

Gay young people have limited role models. They may hide their identity due to peer group pressure. They commonly experience loneliness, isolation and difficulties making contact with other gay people (Plummer, 1995). In the case of working-class youths who have limited formal education, this could prove even more difficult. Involvement in further and higher education leads to the development of many skills, including the ability to gain access to information. The emergence of gay and lesbian organisations and incentives, such as the gay switchboard during the 1980s, helped to lessen the trauma of the 'coming out' process (Plummer, *op cit*). Nevertheless, 'coming out' can still be very difficult, not least because of the variety of responses a gay or lesbian person might encounter. Discovery that their son or daughter is gay may initiate grief in parents. They will need to relinquish other hopes and assumptions, for example, that they might one day become grandparents (Markowe, *op cit*). Markowe distinguishes between 'coming out to self', and 'coming out to others' summarising these as two associated, but nevertheless independent processes. Another of the participants recalls:

> It is difficult, because on the one hand you have to face up to the fact that you might be gay. Like, you start to realise that other fellas sort of 'turn you on' and that the idea of having sex with a woman is somehow, well, I don't know, 'not right'. Me, I thought it was just a phase to be honest, some of the books tell you that don't they? So I did have a few sexual relationships with girls, but it never felt right... I finally admitted to myself that I must be gay... that was bad enough... but then I had to face up to telling people, especially my family... that was really hard, especially with my parents, because they have never accepted it. I don't blame them to be honest, I did then, when I was younger. But I think now I'm old enough to appreciate that

> it must be very hard. I mean, the thing is, my parents weren't what you might call 'homophobic' not at all. Yet they couldn't accept it in their own son.

Coming out to colleagues at work presents different problems. Some of the lesbians who took part in Markowe's study decided against 'coming out' at work because they assumed that they might be vulnerable to discrimination. All three of the gay men interviewed had 'come out' at work, although at different periods in their lives. Two 'came out' altogether (told everyone they knew, as soon as they had made the decision to come out). The third 'came out' in his thirties, after spending many years hiding his identity from significant others. Social class was one of the reasons he gave for this:

> I think that, for the more middle-class gay, they can pick and choose to a certain extent where they live. I do think it is fair to say that it's more acceptable, being gay in some areas than others. But where I lived, it was dog rough, I mean, you just don't take risks like, your reputation when you came out as gay, you risked life and limb. I mean, they would beat the shit out of you where I come from... I mean, after I did come out, there was the AIDs scare, and I was coming home to find spray paint on the front door, the garage door. I mean, it's not safe in an area like that to come out.

'Coming out' is not a 'one off' a 'once and for all' act. It is a continuous process. At work, as old colleagues leave, new colleagues begin. Over time, responses to each 'coming out' can be very different. Sometimes people 'come out' themselves, at other times people hear about the gay person via gossip. One of the gay men interviewed was rather amused by some of the responses he had encountered during his working life:

> One guy just could not believe it. He kept walking past me and staring at me. Then he got some of his friends to come with him while he stared at me. I just ignored it, until he started walking past me with a mate and pointing at me, with a real look of loathing and disapproval in his face. Then I raised the roof and do you know, I wonder sometimes are people 'thick'? Or do they just act that way to get out of trouble? I mean, when I pointed out that that kind of behaviour was harassment, he just, well he seemed genuinely surprised and upset... I mean, he seemed really genuine... I think that's part of the trouble really. That, if a person is different, in any way, there is this assumption that ordinary things will not offend... and I'm sorry, but all this politeness, and assertiveness lark. The only way to

> bring it home to people like that is to act outraged... to really raise the bloody roof and make it very clear that that kind of behaviour is not acceptable. Acting polite, that's letting them win, letting them think you are different, that you need their permission to be treated like a human being — sod that for a tale!

However, despite having recalled some pretty painful experiences, two of the three men denied ever having considered suicide.[14] The one who had experienced depression did not relate this to his gayness, but rather to other life traumas. This participant admitted a tendency to develop episodes of clinical depression from time to time. So it seems that homosexual identity, despite any discrimination experienced, is not, in itself sufficient to lead to suicidal thoughts. Can the experience of 'coming out', no matter how problematic, also lead to positive outcomes? And can these provide a 'buffer' against other traumas? Is secrecy, the need to hide, one predisposing factor? One of the participants interviewed discussed a relative of hers who had openly identified himself as a transvestite in the last year of his life. She noted that 'he was very guilty about this, of course he tried to hide it'.

A year after 'coming out' as a transvestite to his family, this man committed suicide. This presents the case of a young man who had been married. For much of his life he had 'passed' as 'normal' in all respects. Some family members, when he came out, rejected him:

> His brother, when he found out, went totally, totally against him... you see it can be hard for people to realise that people are not always as they would like them to be, I mean, in Xs case, he wasn't as masculine as they [his family] would have liked him to be. He had this feminine side, that was very, very strong, and he had a real need to express it, but that can be very hard for people to understand.[15]

But was this man's suicide solely due to rejection? The transcript material suggests a much more complex picture than this. Indeed, this and all of the stories collected for this study suggest the

14 From a theoretical perspective this is interesting because the men's stories did include many accounts that might predispose many people to consider suicide. This included feelings of stigma, identity crisis, loneliness, deep feelings of unhappiness and isolation. This finding does not, of course, invalidate previous research, but it does draw attention to the complexity and multi factorial nature of suicidal risk and, indeed, immunity.

15 Relative of a man who committed suicide (age withheld) he did not report ever having suicidal thoughts.

accumulation of a multitude of factors before the suicide took place. So, although sexual identity may be one contributing factor, this alone is unlikely to lead to suicide. Identity confusion is partly attributable to physiological changes that are occurring. It is not the physical changes alone that cause conflict. Acceptance by one's peers seems very important. Sexuality and sexual identity are clearly important here, but this is only a part of the process of the adult maturity required to make long-term commitments. Group membership, acceptance and a sense of belonging are a part of this. These can be established in a variety of contexts.

Religion, group membership and 'belonging'

One of the participants, who took part in this study, remarked on the horrifying numbers of people that are homeless, or living alone in bed-sits. She observed that many are lonely and isolated. Sometimes, young people seek emotional asylum by absorbing themselves in political ideologies, beliefs or causes. Sometimes this provides a sense of identity and belonging. The Spiritualist Church in the town of Bolton, for example, attracts a great many young, otherwise lonely people. As one participant put it 'they say that they don't fit in, but they fit in here'. Religious faith can protect people from developing suicidal thoughts (Durkheim, 1952). Parkes *et al* (1997) write that the word 'religion' comes from the Latin word 'reiagare' meaning 'to bind'. 'To bind' is an emotionally loaded term. To 'be bound' can be comforting, a reminder of the security of infancy, but it can also be tyrannical, oppressive and restricting. Relating the term 'to bind' to religion, Parkes and Blanche also note that religion needs to have a degree of flexibility. If religion fails to meet the needs of the people (whatever these needs may be) then people will abandon it, or seek alternatives. Kenny (1998a) drawing on the work of Dale (1985) noted that as the orthodox religious institutions in the town of Bolton became more middle-class, working-class people began to move away from them. However, less orthodox religions, such as spiritualism, are becoming increasingly popular in the town, particularly among the young. This research suggests that it appears to be the perceived unconditional that draws young people to the Spiritualist Church:[16]

16 When compared to the perceived lack of acceptance of the more orthodox churches.

> I find it quite worrying now, the number of young people who come here, the number who say that they feel like doing it, the number who are doing it — much more than older people, or so it seems to me. Because no matter how depressed a person of around fifty or sixty might be, they have the confidence to be at home with themselves. Young people today, so many are struggling to feel 'whole'. I think it's a reflection of the times that we are living in. All the old communities are gone now, or are breaking down. The schools are massive, they are over-crowded. The doctors are busy, the teachers are busy, even parents are busy. People are getting increasingly wary about getting involved. The end result is that we have a great many young people that are lost and desperate, they can find no one who will listen. And yet they drift in here, sometimes I think they are just curious, or maybe they just want to get warm, get a cup of tea or whatever. But then they decide that they like it here, and they start to attend quite regularly. I think part of it might be company, but here, at the church, we try to encourage people, especially younger people, to think about their worth. When they first start to get involved, at our meetings, I will often ask them 'what is your value?' It's surprising how many find it hard at first to answer that, but they do eventually, start to look at themselves, and to find some value in what they have to offer.[17]

This account suggests that this particular church at least, adopts an open, accommodating and accepting approach. There appears to be an assumption that everyone has certain talents, certain 'gifts' to offer. In recent years, psychologists have been taking an increasing interest in the role of religion in promoting good emotional, physical and mental health. It seems that religion can give people hope, a sense of continuity, of belonging and social support. However, religion and social support share the potential to breed dependency, uncertainty and lack of confidence (Burleson *et al*, 1994). Participants considered that many young people who attend the Spiritualist Church feel let down by 'the system', especially schools. Many of the town's 'better' schools are religious establishments, from which some of the young people who took part in this study had been excluded. The participants were alert to the problems that exclusion from school can lead to. A youth worker interviewed, observed that exclusion can have long-term negative effects. He also acknowledged some of the problems faced by teachers and social workers who try to help young

17 Female participant aged around 55–60 years of age.

people. It is assumed that we now live in a classless society, but the participant above makes the interesting assertion that class barriers were perhaps less important, and more 'crossable' in the recent past. This he attributes to the barriers having been more explicit. The pressures on middle-class professional people were less intense:

> I don't think that a lot of young people today have the necessary skills and confidence [to make a meaningful life for themselves] if you see what I mean. Say you come from a working-class back ground. I mean some of the working- class areas around here, well all of the parents are unemployed never mind the children. Well, the kids, they have no forward view of things, they have no respect for themselves or for anyone else, their parents, their schools, they have all talked down to them. So it just carries on and carries on... and I mean, there are limits to how much professional people can help young people from those kinds of backgrounds. I'm not being awful, but no matter how nice they are, and I mean, even if they 'dress down' so to speak, the minute they open their mouths, their whole manner is middle-class. How much can a person like that relate to some of the young people who are having problems in a place like Bolton? I mean, what do they really understand about what many of the working-class families around here have to do to survive? What can they teach the kids about how to survive in that kind of environment? I mean, a lot of these social workers, they are like teachers really. They are just another authority figure to many of these kids... I feel sorry for the teachers, I'm not blaming them because many of these schools are massive. When I went to school, there were 500 kids in that school all told. I don't think social class actually mattered that much then, because the teachers knew the kids. They had to spend less time accounting for themselves and more time getting to know the kids and their families. Now! They don't know the kids, and its all this meeting targets. It must be very frustrating for them, it must be very hard to feel that they are achieving anything in Bolton at the moment. Heroin is rife. It really is mind blowing, unbelievable how it has grown in the last seven or eight years. I don't know! And it's trying to understand why, so many young people get lost like that.[18]

Establishments, such as religious ones and the school, can provide a sense of belonging and group membership for some young people,

18 32-year-old male participant — has attempted and considered suicide during his adolescent years (age not specified) but not in recent years.

but not all. If a young person finds it difficult, for whatever reason, to establish their membership of a more 'socially accepted' group, they may search for other contexts in which they might establish their identity. Membership of an 'out group' (no matter how deviant) offers one route to group membership. In Bolton there is a rising drugs problem. The participant observes that many of the town's heroin addicts had been excluded from socially legitimate contexts, such as the school. In the next section we consider deviance and risk behaviour.

Risk behaviour, deviance and group membership

Identities are not unchanging. They shift, reflecting our changing life contexts (Hunt and Robbins, 1998). We also have more than one identity and our self-esteem and sense of worth fluctuates, depending on which identity is expressed at any given time. Identities that are negative are 'off balanced' by those that are more positive. Positive or negative identity is as much an experiential as a socially determined thing. We form our identifications according to our group membership. Membership of a group considered 'deviant' can establish a positive sense of worth, if members of that group value each other. This is why it is very wrong to assume that members of 'out groups' necessarily have low self-esteem. Quite the contrary, membership of the out group may be the only source of positive worth that some people have.[19] Group membership can be established by participating in work, hobbies, or relationships. What we do is a very important part of who we are. If we write, paint, bring up children, teach, or have no socially approved pastime, eg. if we are unemployed, all of these things help us define what we are. Membership of a deviant group may offer the only means available for a young person, who lacks confidence, to find some sense of worth (Burt, 1969). Unfortunately, in making such affiliations they establish a negative reputation that is hard to relinquish. Young people who associate with socially accepted groups distance themselves (understandably) and this makes rehabilitation difficult. If the boundaries that separate groups appear too difficult to reconcile, then people are inclined to tighten them (Tajfel, 1978).

Young people can be so concerned about what and who they are

19 This discussion is developed further in the section on risk behaviour.

that 'in group' acceptance becomes very important to them. This at least offers some sense of security. But sometimes, life brings experiences that mitigate against a young person ever developing a sense of belonging. A young participant who had spent time (three months) in a young offenders institution recalls his sense of desolation when he came back to his local community:

> I think that it was then that it came home to me that you have to share, sort of thing, to belong. I mean, I remember that I cried myself to sleep about this for weeks and weeks. Like, I thought I could just come back home and everything would be the same, that I'd just carry on with my mates like I had always done. But we'd be out and, they'd be going on about things that had happened while I was away, things they knew all about and it was like, news to me. I really felt out of it. But I was lucky, my mates were pretty good... they did do their best to make me feel accepted, and after a time it was all right. But yes, I can understand how people might get suicidal in a situation like that, I mean, I really felt the most terrible, awful sense of loneliness... far more than when I went in [to the institution] 'cos in there, so long as you get your respect,[20] you can be all right.[21]

In order to protect their own sense of positive worth, children and young people can be very cruel, even at times, excluding members of their own group. In the young offenders institution, for example, it is the 'muppets' (those who fail to get their 'respect') who apparently suffer the most discrimination. To be a member, even if placed on the margins of an 'outsider' group, is (no matter how isolating or discriminatory) an identity of a kind. Characterising adolescence as a time when most young people 'start to learn about the world in earnest' the Royal College of Psychiatrists (1998a) argues that they 'crave excitement in a way that most adults find difficult to understand'. Adolescence is also a time when young people engage in high levels of risk behaviour, a kind of 'flirting with death' that some writers put down to their increased awareness of their own

20 The young man referred to 'getting your respect' several times during his interview. When I enquired what this meant, he explained that young men (and possibly young women) need to establish their 'toughness' in order to be accepted by their peers in such institutions. How this was done, the young man was reluctant to discuss, but he did refer to 'muppets' that is, young people who did not get their respect, who needed to survive by obliging other inmates by the completion of certain tasks, such as cleaning shoes and handing over cigarettes etc.

21 A 23-year-old who man reported suicidal thoughts from time to time, but no attempts.

mortality (Kastenbaum, 1986). Substance dependency is becoming a major concern for many parents. Injection or inhalation of opiates, such as heroin, cause powerful euphoric feelings of warmth and relaxation. However, tolerance to and dependency on such drugs can develop within weeks. Abrupt withdrawal can lead to withdrawal symptoms (Beard, 1995). Health education may have a limited role to play, but it seems that many of the young people who are involved in drugs are well aware of the dangers. While acknowledging that 'the roots of suicidal behaviour lie in many different social, health and educational problems', Rioch (*op cit*) also notes the recommendations that, 'suicide prevention should include the self-destructive behaviours of substance abuse and eating disorders'.

The targets outlined in the *Health of the Nation* document (DoH, 1992) aim to reduce the number of deaths caused by risk behaviours that are directly or indirectly caused by drug use. These targets aim to, 'reduce the overall suicide by 15%, the number of accidental deaths in people aged between 15–20 years by 25% and, in relation to HIV and AIDs, to reduce by 50% the numbers of injecting drug users who report sharing needles' (McKie, 1994). However, the *Health of the Nation* has been criticised for a number of reasons, including its individualism and the assumption that providing information alone is sufficient to change behaviour (Naidoo and Wills, 1994; Mackintosh, 1996; McKie, *op cit*). As the extract below suggests, the picture is much more complex than this:

> But that is why it is such a serious problem [the deaths of peers does not appear to be a deterrent]. The only thing that matters, nothing matters, you don't matter, nobody matters. And in a daft kind of way it gives them something to do. They have to find the heroin, they have to find the means to pay for the heroin. There's like, a whole culture attached to it really... at least it's something to live for, you know what I mean. It becomes a whole way of life for them, it gives them something to do. I mean, in some ways it can be a good life. I know that sounds daft, but at least they are part of something, and the problem is it excludes taking advantage of anything else. I know people who have tried to get off it, once, twice maybe even three or four times. But they can't get accepted, it goes against them, the fact that they have been on it. So they start again and go back to the group where they can be accepted. I mean, it's the system, the whole system has failed them.[22]

22 Man in his thirties, discussing drug addition, has not considered suicide, but has lost a family member due to drug addition.

One of the funeral directors interviewed observed that many drug addicts in the town attend the funerals of friends who have died of overdoses. Following the service, these young people can be observed around the side of the church 'shooting'. Freud believed that there was a suicidal thread in us all. Shneidman (1963) refers to 'sub-intentional deaths', ie. those that do not appear to be directly due to a suicide. Such deaths are neither clearly suicidal, accidental nor natural. What happens in such cases is that the deceased had played an unconscious role in permitting his or her own death (Freud, 1901/1974, cited by Wass, 1995; Shneidman, 1963; Murry, 1967). 'The very lifestyles of some people appears to demean their lives to the point where they are as good as dead' (Leenaars, 1995). Freud (1901/1974, cited by Wass, 1995) suggested that severe cases of self-injury may often suggest symptoms of this phenomena, including some (apparently) accidental injuries. Sub-intentional injury is also common in sufferers of post-traumatic stress disorder (Kenny, 1998b). Such individuals may not be aware that they wish to kill themselves, but, as one funeral director suggested, they are, in effect, as good as dead.[23]

It would need further research to establish whether such an apparently blatant disregard of the dangers is due to some kind of desire to 'self-destruct'. However, the limited material gathered for this book suggests that it is more a need for acceptance, more a case of finding something to do, that motivates much of the drug-related behaviour, at least in the town. In other words, it appears that there is much more going on here than the need for a 'kick'. Drug dependency in this context is not an individual, but rather a collective and relational phenomenon. If we want to understand relationships, what makes or breaks them, then we have to understand the meaning that people assign to them (Duck, 1994; Miell and Dallos, 1996). In relation to the extract above it appears that being part of the 'drug culture' gives some young people a sense of belonging, group membership and, as the participant above notes, it gives young people something to do. Life as a heroin addict is active not passive.

23 Other forms of indirect suicide include martyrdom, neurotic individualism, alcohol addiction, anti-social behaviour and psychosis. In all of these conditions, the person places themselves at risk. 'Focal suicide' refers to self-mutilation, often of a specific body part. This self-mutilating may not be direct, it can be expressed, for example, in multiple surgery, purposive accidents, impotence and frigidity. Suicide can also have an organic component, focusing on the psychological factors involved in the vent of an organic disease, especially the self-punishing, aggressive and erotic components. (For a more detailed discussion, see Wass, 1995.)

Planning how to get the drug, planning how to pay for it, provides meaning, purpose and structure to the day. For those who have more attractive alternatives, this must appear a very negative existence, but it is an existence of a kind, and better than no kind.

The term 'risk' currently suggests a negative health outcome. However, those who are taking the risks may see things in terms of probability rather than certainty. Individuals may be aware of the health risks involved in their behaviour, but there may be positive aspects attached to the risk behaviour that overrule any perceived negatives (Mackintosh, 1996). Finally, in relation to information giving, and support, McKie observes that, 'the number of groups that a young person comes into contact with, the nature of support provision, reflects the social and economic characteristic of the household, the locality and the region', and that, 'given the target of reducing suicide, which is more prevalent amongst young men, may require societal change to address employment and social roles'. In *Chapter 3* we discuss the role of health education and promotion in relation to mental health, risk behaviour and suicide. For the present discussion, it seems sufficient to end with the observation that, for many young drug users, it will take more than the provision of information to address the problem. As long as it appears to some young people, that life involved with the 'drugs scene' has more to offer then anything else, it seems unlikely that this particular form of risk behaviour will be reduced. However, would meaningful employment for all solve the problem?

Employment, youth and identity

As adolescence proceeds, adulthood looms increasingly near. A young person may fear that he/she will fail to live up to other people's expectations. Three of the participants who took part in this study made worrying observations of the pressure young people experience to do well academically. They also noted the diversity of youth experience, ie. that while some young people may feel overwhelmed by the numerous opportunities open to them, others might feel restricted and 'hemmed in' by how few they have available to them. Some of the participants also remarked on the importance of factors, such as education, culture, gender and social class in shaping such opportunities (or indeed, the lack of them). In many respects, post-modernity has created difficulties for young people, both restricting and at the same time limiting their ability to secure any consistent sense of identity. The world has become a much more unstable and unpredictable place (Frosh, 1991; Giddens, 1991; Woodward, 1997). Long-term planning of life, love and career has become far more tentative and insecure:

> These days, an awful lot of young people, especially those between 18 and 20 years old, they don't feel that they belong, they have no goal and there is terrible widespread loneliness. There is a tendency to think that if a person is young they should not be lonely, that they will have lots of friends, but it's not like that. I mean, let's face it, loneliness is not the same as being alone, and if there is no way, I mean work, having a family, feeling 'normal' for want of a better word, then a young person has as much, maybe more chance of being lonely than an older person. This comes up time and time again, I mean, there are a lot of young people around here living in bed-sits, or homeless even. How can they have any sense of belonging if they have nowhere to live, or if where they live, there is no sense of community... these bed-sits can be very isolated you know. I think its due to a variety of reasons really, I mean, you can't just walk into a job these days, even if you have all these qualifications... and even the most menial of work can give people a sense of worth and a sense of purpose. I mean, for all they may have been menial in many ways, many of the old apprentices, even the boring mundane jobs did at least give young people a sense of belonging, some sense of pride.

Here the participant discusses the problem of homelessness in the young. If identity is connected to stability, to a sense of 'belonging' in the locational as well as spiritual sense, then clearly homelessness will confound any ambition to develop any positive sense of self. The participant also touches on the issue of unemployment, a problem that often contributes to homelessness. Unemployment severely restricts a person's ability to choose where and how they live. Many of the young unemployed may be separated from their families. They may be homeless, or live in the more 'undesirable' areas. The negative effects of slum environments on self-esteem, crime and delinquency was explored by Conant (1962). This study, and many others have shown how negative environments, such as slum areas, can lead to feelings of powerlessness, depression and ill health (Seligman, 1975; Gilbert, 1992). In the nineties it would be comforting to assume that things have improved. In fact, inequalities in health due to issues, such as gender, class and ethnicity, are still very much a reality (Whitehead, 1987). Some voluntary organisations, such as MIND and CRISIS are very energetic and committed to addressing homelessness, hunger and poverty. The solutions (although very helpful in practical terms) are based on Victorian charitable values, which (no matter how unintended) can be very demeaning to recipients. If we relate this to our discussion of the development of identity, this kind of 'soup kitchen' approach is unlikely to promote positive self-esteem. Commenting on the high rates of unemployment and the effect that this can have on self-esteem, Rioch (1994) argues that young people should be encouraged to find 'new ways of living a meaningful life in the absence of work'. Spending time waiting for your local charities weekly street distribution of food and clothing could hardly be interpreted as a 'meaningful' existence. She further argues that young people should 'find ways of investing themselves, without a loss of self-worth, towards a future that may be different from their expectations of a life of full-time employment'.[24] This is difficult for a young person in a society that adopts a very punitive attitude towards unemployment. Another participant discussed how humiliating experiences at the unemployment/social security office could be:

> A lot of the whole approach these days is to be 'professional', to be sort of detached and to put a distance between 'them', the unemployed that is, and 'us' that's 'us' who have a proper job. The thing is, there is many a young person who comes here, really demoralised because of the kind of snotty attitude that they have to deal with at those places, and its approved of, you know. And every effort seems to be put on doing them out of as many benefits as possible and for punishing them, it's a kind of brainwashing really, against daring to think that they are of any worth at all... like, if they appear too demanding or they dare to speak out say, about having to wait too long. These are young people who already have a really low sense of worth, and some people should never be put in a position of power you know? I really truly believe that. They seem to take a real pride in belittling a lot of these young people, and I often think, 'oh, if only you could spare a thought for what you are doing to them', but you see, some people are incapable of that, because their self-worth is dependent on other people being belittled.[25]

24 The author wishes to stress that she greatly admires the work of the organisations discussed above (at least they are doing something). The comments above should be interpreted in the context in which they are made, that is, the effects that being a recipient of charity may have on self-esteem.

25 Woman aged around 60 years of age.

The narrative above begins with an assumption that it is unemployment that causes youth unhappiness, but as the speaker continues, it becomes clear that it is not so much unemployment that leads to a lack of self-worth, but rather the way that unemployed people are treated. Traditional psychology does embrace the notion that work (especially if this includes involvement with a good mentor) is a valuable source of positive self-worth. Work also offers a means to establish an identity, but we need to distinguish between the unemployed who have lost their jobs and the young unemployed who have never had a job. A recent study showed that older people who had been made redundant had less negative attitudes towards unemployment than younger people. This was because younger people with little employment experience were more likely to idealise work. Older people, however, had a much more cynical view of it, and were more concerned with the financial aspects of unemployment than they were with concerns about threats to identity (Breakwell, 1996).

Work can be boring, soul-destroying and monotonous, as a study conducted by the author in 1994 of northern women's experiences of the textile industry demonstrated. Some textile workers actually hated working in the cotton mills. Without wishing to devalue the benefits of work, the assumption that solving youth unemployment (assuming that this could be done) would necessarily lead to a significant reduction in youth unhappiness and suicide is questionable. The Protestant work ethic is still influential, making it all too easy to assume that paid employment is always beneficial whereas unemployment is always deleterious to health. The January 1999 edition of *The Psychologist* presents a collection of papers that outline some of the negative and emotionally distressing aspects of paid employment, while the editorial contains a commentary on the current high rates of stress in workers, especially those employed in the public sector.[26] It is mistaken to assume that work is always fulfilling, always a source of positive worth, always meaningful and productive. O'Connell (1995) reminds us of earlier, wealthier generations who had no need to work and did not do so and observes that few appeared unhappy 'probably because they had never heard of the Protestant work ethic'. Argle (1992) identifies income as one of the variables that significantly increases (although it does not guarantee) happiness. So, is solving unemployment necessarily the answer to reducing youth unhappiness and suicide?

26 *The Psychologist*, January 1999, **12**(1).

One of the participants who took part in this study for example, argued that it is not so much unemployment that is the problem, but the way that technology has been implemented. Rather than have two groups, that is 'the out of work and the worked to death' why should not everyone benefit from technology; with part-time work and reasonable wages for all? Is a return to full employment unlikely as Boyle (1991) suggests? If so, should we consider the possibility of introducing a minimum income. According to Boyle (1998) part of the problem stems from the way that Western society values only paid employment. Other forms of work, for example, child minding, decorating the house and general community activities, such as those fulfilled by the voluntary sector, are officially considered 'unproductive'. Perhaps the solution might be to introduce an unconditional minimum income for every individual. This would 'attack poverty by providing an income on which people with low earnings' potential could build through work and savings' (Citizens Income Study Centre, 1998). Would having a reasonable income in itself, give people a sense of purpose. There is insufficient scope to discuss this issue in depth in this text. It does seem that it is becoming increasingly unreasonable and unrealistic to educate young people in such a way that they learn to expect paid employment in adult life. As Rioch (*op cit*) suggests, it might be more useful to teach young people alternative ways of giving meaning to their lives, without work. If such an approach develops in education, then we need to also refrain from punishing people if they do not find work. We also need to find some way of facilitating the development of a 'meaningful life' (whatever that may be). Currently, there are young people of around 19 to 20 years of age, who left school early, have never had a job and have been 'unproductive' for approximately five years. Such young people may need to be rehabilitated in order to develop purpose and structure to their days. There was a time when the author considered calls for the reintroduction of national service with caution, but in recent years, observations have led her to consider that a voluntary period spent in a similar, structured and supportive environment (following which, there might be a gradual and supported introduction into the community) may actually prove useful for some young people. Some of the aims of such an environment would include support and the teaching of life and social skills. Such arrangements might ease the transition to adulthood and reduce some of the anxiety associated with separation. Who knows? There may come a time when it proves useful to introduce 'social service' instead of 'national service'.

If young people establish a positive identity, they proceed to the stage of intimacy, followed by that of generativity. Generativity is a creative term and refers not just to the raising of children, but also the production of work and ideas. For young working-class people finding a source of independent (and for them) creative productive work can be difficult. They might resort to finding ways to survive outside 'official' systems. This approach has a long and deeply established history in some working-class communities and is linked partly to ideas about what counts as a valued existence and partly, perhaps, because of a suspicion of all things related to bureaucracy, 'the system' and class boundaries. The young man cited below comments in his observations on changing patterns of labour. He notes that workers have become more vulnerable in all social classes, but the meaning and consequences in different cases are different:

> I mean, I don't think that all this lack of security helps, and it's the same for everyone, even people like yourself who are working in universities, many of them are on short-term contracts, two or three years here, another two or three years there. I mean, for the working-class, especially in things like the building trade, its always been like that. Some work here, some work there. It's a free and easy life really, or rather it was, and one that, despite all the insecurities, people could enjoy. You know, there was enough for a drink in the pub with the lads, and a fairly comfortable lifestyle and a kind of acceptance. But the wages when you had them were OK, you knew they would cover you for the times in between [jobs]. But that was OK when work was pretty well paid and in abundance. But what was lacking was this deferred gratification. There wasn't the need for that then, but the kids need it now because things have changed. It's harder now to make a little bit here, and a little bit there... live a kind of easy lifestyle, more or less living off your wits, living day-to-day with a very general sort of acceptance of what each day brings. I mean, that way of life, its had it now. And most working-class parents have grown up with it, so they haven't taught their children the importance of this deferred gratification thing, they never learned it for themselves, so they never taught it to their kids. So everyone I suppose is at a bit of a loss. Those who used to be able to think long-term, they can't really plan anymore for more than two or three years. Whereas, those who had learned to live day to day, they can't manage by the old ways because things have tightened up. I mean, you can't win. Whether you try to look long-term or short-term, the result's the same. No security. No hope of security.

The same participant later in the discussion cites the case of some young people who had attempted to adopt a kind of 'self-sufficiency' outside the 'system'. As he notes, despite the rhetoric in favour of 'self-sufficiency' that is so prevalent today, it is only accepted within formal structures:

> I know young lads, they are 16 and they have just left school. They tried to make a little extra cash, like, cash in hand like, doing people's gardens like. They were only charging a fiver and they were doing a really good job of it. But then someone squealed on them... well how can you be so peevish like. I mean, so they were playing the system a little, but maybe they needed to for a while, just until they got a bit of something behind them. And who knows they might have really built something. But people are peevish now. Whereas they might have turned a blind eye to it a few years ago, and maybe think, well here are a couple of young people who are showing a little incentive, trying to build something, they 'shopped' them.

The participant also draws attention not just to changing values, but also to changing patterns of labour. The increase in developments in technology has led to a change from heavy to light industry. This has led to more people becoming labelled as having a learning disability. One man for example, made the following observations:

> My dad was a builder. He was involved in the building trade and he had a really good job. He was well paid and we had a pretty good standard of living. Well, one day I had been off school, I had been ill. When my dad came home, my mum had nipped out, and I remembered that I needed a note to take to school, so I asked my dad to write me one. He said 'sorry son, you'll have to ask your mam to do that'. And then it began to dawn on me, various things like, he always managed to get out of helping me with my homework. He'd encourage me, but he always had a good excuse for getting out of actually helping me. As I got older I began to realise that he had problems with reading, spelling and all this. Now today, he'd be out of a job, unemployable. People would call him 'thick' probably, he'd be labelled as having a learning difficulty. But it didn't matter then, because he was a bloody good tradesman, he had respect for everyone and he had all the things that 'normal' people have, you know, a home, a job, a family.[27]

The participant cited above noted that more people are likely to be classified as having a learning disability at the present time. He also

27 Man in his early forties, has never considered suicide.

draws attention to the fact that people who have literacy problems may find it difficult, if not impossible, to help their children complete homework. This means, given the current focus on parental responsibility, that the problem may be perpetuated from one generation to another. As the participant also noted indirectly, becoming labelled in this way can cut off other possibilities that are a part of adult status. People who have a learning disability may be at particular risk of becoming suicidal. Much of the distress that they suffer may be socially created, rather than a product of individual 'dysfunction'. As the need to gain experience of both further and higher education increases, people who have a learning disability may be at greater risk of becoming socially disadvantaged. They have fewer opportunities to gain affluent status and all of the trappings that go with it, ie. employment, good housing and so forth. However, much of this will depend on the degree of negotiation involved in the labelling process. Labels can be useful and empowering if they identify a problem that can be managed and explain what had once seemed 'inexplicable', forming a basis for self-definition.

Learning difficulties can limit a person's life in a variety of ways. It reduces a person's ability to maintain an active social life. Literacy problems can make it very hard for a person to conduct the most basic tasks connected with social life. Attending a social event, for example, requires the ability to write a confirmation that one is attending. It requires the ability to plan a journey, establish a route, to time the journey, work out public transport schedules and so forth. These are important considerations given that the ability to be able to travel to maintain relationships, may depend on a person's literacy skills. For an increasing number of young people, the ability to actually develop something for themselves, to take some responsibility for others, is reducing. And all this at a time when more opportunities appear to be available than ever before.

Conclusion

This chapter has explored how progression through Erkison's stages presents conflicts and challenges as the young person struggles to gain some sense of identity. The accomplishment of earlier tasks, such as trust, is important, but adolescence and young adulthood can be a traumatic time influenced by potential threats to identity, such as separation, employment and the need to belong. If young people are unable to establish themselves in the more socially accepted groups, then they may be vulnerable to risks and possibly deviance. If the challenges prove too much, too isolating, then suicide may seem the only solution. The concept of generativity assumes a level of maturity in which people are able to take responsibility for others, put the needs of other's before themselves and to make commitments to things, such as a family and a career. Changing patterns of labour and instability, may mitigate against the achievement of Erikson's tasks. Does this necessarily mean that we can expect only hopelessness for young people? Does it mean that society has to change? Or is it that we need to revisit traditional theories in psychology? Do we need to deconstruct them, examine these theories before 'repacking' them in such a way that more historically appropriate stages of adult development are proposed? Until recently, the emphasis in social science has been on deconstruction — which leaves nothing but a lot of confusing, disorientated 'pieces'. We need more than this if we are to address the problem of suicide and young people.

3

The promotion of mental health and the prevention of suicide

Introduction

The increase in attempted and completed suicide in the young is clearly a cause for concern. Research suggests that (and this is perhaps the greatest tragedy) many acts of suicide may have been preventable. Many people who commit suicide do want to live, but they feel unable to conceive of any solutions to their dilemmas. Suicidal people often give warnings that others do not recognise (the Samaritans, 1998). Surviving family members not only suffer the trauma of bereavement, but are themselves at greater risk of committing suicide (Wertheimer, 1991; Hahn, 1998). In *The Drowned and the Saved,* the survivor, Levi (1986), wrote that suicide was rare in the concentration camps during World War II. He suggests three possible explanations for this. First, he observes that an act of suicide implies an element of choice. People who lived in the concentration camps had no choices. They lived in constant danger of being killed by others, but unable to kill themselves. Second, the camps nurtured a survival culture in which people had no time to think about suicide. Third, having observed that guilt can be the cause of many suicide attempts, he argued that those in the concentration camps felt that they were being punished already.[1] Levi's analysis (and indeed, his biography) illustrates the complexity of suicide. It shows that, on the one hand people will struggle to survive, even in the most harrowing circumstances. Yet in other more (seemingly) hopeful and indeed affluent situations, suicide rates can be very high. Levi's observations also bring home the importance of subjective interpretation (what people make of a given situation). We have argued throughout that suicide needs to be understood in relation to social context, but clearly, no matter what the context or situation, individual interpretation, and the methods that individuals develop to

1 Levi committed suicide shortly after the publication of his book. Some have argued that this was due to survival guilt, but the argument that it was probably due to a combination of factors appears more convincing (Dominian, *op cit*).

cope with this, are important. In this chapter we discuss the role of health education and promotion in relation to suicide prevention.

Health education, promotion and the *Health of the Nation*

The priorities outlined in the *Health of the Nation* (1992) include the promotion of mental health and of strategies aimed at reducing suicide. The document also includes a stated commitment to reducing risk behaviours that contribute towards premature deaths. The document has been heavily criticised. McKie (1994) comments on the emphasis on bringing about behavioural change alongside an absence of any discussion for how such change is best brought about. Following Akenhurst *et al* (1991) she suggests that target setting will inevitably fail if it is based on 'unclear selection criteria, unclear strategies for how these are to be achieved, and an unwillingness to devote resources so that these might be realised'. Following Ingledrew (1989), she notes that it overlooks health determinants that exist outside the individual's control.

It is clear that health promotion and education have a crucial role to play in suicide prevention. The terms health promotion and health education are often used interchangeably, although Mackintosh (1996) argues that this is misleading. Differences between the two need to be explored before the discussion proceeds. Following Dennis *et al* (1982), Mackintosh defines health promotion as a diverse, broad, large scale project that 'covers all aspects of those activities that seek to improve the health status of individuals and communities'. McKie (1994) charts the field of health promotion as having evolved alongside a growing support for the public health movement, which emerged due to increasing awareness of the complex variables that combine to influence people's health. She writes, 'health promotion can be defined as any planned activity which enhances health or prevents disease. It encompasses screening, education and general promotion activities'. Health promotion is 'an approach to health care which, by necessity, incorporates a political dimension and an awareness of the power dynamic which can characterise interactions between health professionals, individuals and communities. It is an approach to health care which, at its best, has a basis for action originating from communities'.

Definitions such as this appear to place health promotion in direct opposition to the values underpinning capitalism. These are fundamentally socialist values that undermine purely utilitarian notions of health, such as concerns to maintain the productive efficiency of the workforce.[2] Jackson's (1988) *Moon Walker* (despite any 'humanistic' values glorified in the film) illustrates all too well, that one must become (literally) a 'man of steel' to survive in such a context. However, there has been an increasing awareness in recent years, of the impact that environmental factors play in relation to health and disability (Naidoo and Wills, 1994; McKie and Mackintosh, *op cit*; Pepper, 1996; Ussher, 1991; Beresford and Wallcraft, 1997; Barnes and Mercer, 1996). Approaches encompassed within the field of health promotion are very diverse. For the sake of simplicity, these can be placed along a continuum ranging from those that are individualistic in approach (eg. the biomedical, educational and behavioural change approaches) to those that place a greater emphasis on social issues (eg. the social change and community involvement approaches). Other models acknowledge the various ways that individual and social factors interact. Some models have a predominantly 'top down' approach (ie. driven from above by professional groups) while others operate from the 'bottom up'.

Health education is based on the (relatively simplistic) assumption that 'information giving to individuals might result in a behaviour change or avoidance of hazard' (McKie, *op cit*). This assumption reflects a misconception that underpinned many early theories of attitude formation and change, ie. the assumption that there exists a clear correspondence between attitude and behaviour. Research has shown other intervening variables are important, such as the existence of barriers, perceived susceptibility and the dominant social norm (Festinger, 1957, Fishbein, 1967; Becker and Mainman, 1975). Following Baric (1985), Mackintosh (*op cit*) defines health education's primary concern to be that of:

> *Raising individual's competence and knowledge about health and illness, about the body and its functions, about prevention and coping; with raising competence and knowledge to use the health care system and to understand its functions; and with raising awareness about social, political and environmental factors that influence health.*

2 Described very briefly, socialist, naturalistic values place nature (including human nature) as the prime source of worth. Capitalism places worth primarily on the value of consumerism, demand and exchange. For a more detailed and sophisticated discussion, see Pepper, 1996.

It is clear then, that health education constitutes a very important part of health promotion and, despite its individualism, care should be taken not to devalue it. Suicide is a complex phenomenon, so that preventative interventions must also be varied and intensive to be effective. The following discussion focuses first on health promotion approaches that adopt a predominantly 'top down' approach with a particular focus on health education. This will be followed by some discussion on how some models of health promotion might be utilised to the promotion of mental health and the reduction of suicide.

Health education

According to Mackintosh (*op cit*) health education aims to improve the knowledge and skills of individuals so that they can make informed decisions about behaviours that influence their health status. However, an approach that focuses solely on the individual immediately poses problems when we relate it to mental health because the person at risk may be unable to recognise, or may feel unable to convey to others, the level of their distress. Wass (1995) writes that:

> *Although much has been written on the topic of suicide it remains a subject obscured by myth and misunderstanding. Still, it is important to develop education and prevention programs for use in both the home and school. Such programs must recognise that suicidal people generally give warnings about their state of mind and that suicidal threats must be taken seriously and dealt with in a forthright manner, that intervention in suicide plans is often an effective permanent treatment, and that suicidal young people can frequently be helped by a combination of physical and psychological treatment.*

The aim of health education in the context of promoting mental health should consider directing information to both individuals and groups. Information can be conveyed on a large scale using various media sources.[3] Alternatively, information can be conveyed on a small scale basis by visiting schools, youth organisations and parent's groups. This is where distinctions between health education

3 For discussion of the role of media in health education, see Naidoo and Wills, 1994.

and promotion become blurred. Much of the discussion in this section, which is based on increasing information and developing skills, could have been equally (and some might argue, more appropriately) included in other sections. The discussion in this section is about information, its nature and content, the various ways that it might be conveyed, in what contexts and to whom it is directed. Young people need to have access to information about the range of support systems available. They also need confidence and encouragement to feel able to turn to these where necessary. Parents, teachers and health care professionals may provide information on how to recognise depressive or suicidal young people, but they may require guidelines on the best supportive strategies to adopt. There is also a need to develop more tolerant attitudes. Although it could be argued that this is best achieved by adopting some of the health promotion approaches discussed in later sections, the transmission of information as a starting point, is still important.

Support services that are specific to young people and mental health, particularly suicide and self-harming behaviour, are varied. They include mental health services, medical services, hospitals, school guidance officers, youth services, police services and other related services, such as alcohol, drug and sexual health services. Churches and religious groups also have members who can provide support (University of Queensland fact sheet, 1998). There are many voluntary services available in the UK, such as the Samaritans and ChildLine, that can give support, especially during a crisis (see *Appendix*). Limiting young people's access to suicide aids (eg. drugs, firearms) is also important, as is educating the public about the variety of such methods (eg. ropes, given that hanging is one of the most common methods used in the case of child suicides). As suicide prevention programmes are relatively new, it is important that they are evaluated to see if they work. This is no easy task and evaluation of suicide prevention at the present time is almost non-existent (Royal College of Psychiatrists, 1998b; Mercy, 1997).

School is another area where children can learn about health, death, suicide and risk. In recent years there has been a call to introduce suicide education as a preventative measure. Wass (*op cit*), considers it more helpful to 'fit' such education into existing courses, such as developmental and health studies, and/or health studies programmes. The inclusion of lifespan development in the curriculum (including the impact that phenomena, such as bereavement and suicide have on individuals and communities) would greatly enhance the quality of many life science-related subjects. Wass further considers that general studies is another subject area that could include death studies, and incorporation of this topic into any subject area can lead to discussion of wider issues and debates, such as coping with life crisis, aggression, violence, hate, tolerance etc. General studies is a very broad subject and discussion of ethical issues could also be included. Methods developed from the work of Kohlberg (1970) for facilitating children's moral development, might also be adopted to include hypothetical dilemmas that explore the issue of suicide.

Child and adolescent psychiatrists need to be alert to suicide risk factors in children under 15 years of age (Pasho, 1998). Leenaars (*op cit*) asserts the importance of increasing the awareness of behavioural cues that indicate suicide risk. These are complex and often indirect. No single predictive behaviour appears to indicate definite suicide risk, but clues are expressed by people in all age groups. The way that these are expressed varies depending on age and numerous other factors. Cognitive clues include rigidity in thinking (or a narrowing of perceived options) and feelings of being overwhelmed or helpless to change a situation. Suicidal people frequently feel 'boxed in', harassed, or unsuccessful. In such cases, the person uses words such as 'always', 'only', 'never' and 'forever' (Leenaars, *op cit*). Such a 'narrow' outlook has an impact on emotional expressions and behaviour. Emotional clues may be indicted by increased and constant expressions of anxiety, agitation or depression (ChildLine, 1998). The person may behave in an uncharacteristic way, for example, a normally quiet and reserved person may become very outgoing and 'loud'. School performance of children/young people may decline and they may begin to give away their possessions. The presence of risk behaviour is also a strong indicator of the presence of suicidal risk (Bernstein, 1998).

The most precarious times for adolescents are during 'rites of passage', such as graduation, anniversaries and birthdays. Many young people commit suicide after a disciplinary crisis, a rejection or humiliation (Bernstein, 1998). Sexual identity is also important. Thirty percent of adolescent suicides are related to sexuality, especially concerns about sexual preference (Kourany, 1987; Youth Crisis, 1998). Although better able to articulate their feelings and concerns, some cases of teenage depression go undetected, often presenting as a variety of physical problems. Teenagers who have anxieties about separation often complain of gastrointestinal symptoms, indicative of underlying depressive illness (Bernstein, 1997). Other conditions that are also indicative of depression may keep the young person off school, sometimes for a considerable length of time. Such physical complaints include: dizziness, stomach problems, back pain, light-headedness, vomiting and menstrual problems. The onset of bodily changes, such as the onset of menstruation in girls and nocturnal emissions in boys, can be very upsetting, particularly given that such changes may also be linked with intense feelings and emotions related to sexual attraction, orientation and anxieties about appearance. The young person may present with headaches, tiredness, lack of enthusiasm and weight loss. Indeed, a depressed person may complain of severe pain in almost any area of the body. The Bernstein study found little association between the severity of symptoms and the amount of time taken off school. There was, however, a strong association between severity of physical symptoms and the severity of the underlying psychological distress. Bernstein concludes by emphasising the importance of parents, school administrators and physicians being aware of the associations between physical and psychological distress. Early detection of depression can lead to early and more successful intervention, and avoids the use of expensive, time-consuming tests. Similar observations have been made by Talley (1998), who noted that many cases of depression are confused with physiological conditions, such as anaemia, vitamin deficiency or sinus headaches. The depressed person may have frequent abdominal pain, may be constipated or suffer from bouts of diarrhoea.

Baume (1996) expresses concern that, despite suicidal young people expressing clear signals of distress, these are not recognised by many people, including professionals. Indeed, it appears that those closer to a situation are least likely to pick up signs, which are obvious to those outside. To anyone who is close to a young person who expresses distress, he advises a combination of direct questions, with an open, listening approach. The difficult thing for anyone who encounters such a situation, is knowing which to adopt and when. Open ended, probing questions are best to begin with, because these help the listener to assess the situation. Questions such as 'I've noticed that you seem pretty low, how bad are you feeling?' convey interest, concern and a desire to know more. If further questioning suggests that the situation may be serious, then the listener is advised to move on to direct questioning. Questions such as, 'Are you thinking of killing yourself?' may seem difficult to adopt, but are of vital importance. A direct question is more likely to get an honest, direct response. If the young person responds by denying any suicidal response, then this provides a good opportunity to give a follow up comment such as 'good, because I'd be lost without you?'

This indicates not only love and concern, but may also encourage the young person to consider the consequences of their actions. The listener should caution that they do not slip into the use of 'shut up' statements such as, 'you're just having a hard day'.

Depressed people may also have difficulty interpreting 'open' questions such as, 'what's the matter?' Often being in a confused state of mind to begin with, the young person may be unable to decide whether the speaker is asking a very general question, or a specific question where the intention is to assess their state of mind. Baume stresses the importance of listeners controlling their own emotions during questioning, and of probing further until a complete assessment (one that satisfies the listener) is achieved. While some problems can be dealt with inside the family, others may be more serious. Where this latter situation is indicated, the listener should not be afraid or reluctant to seek help, or to encourage the speaker to do so. Sometimes, offering to accompany a distressed young person may provide greater encouragement.

The traditional notion that it is dangerous to discuss suicide with depressed young people, because of the assumption that such a discussion might lead to it, has been replaced with a recommendation that children should be encouraged to discuss all their feelings, including any suicidal feelings that they may have. Wass recommends that direct questions designed to discover how the young person is feeling should be phrased in a supportive, non-judgemental way. There is also a need to be direct and clear about concerns. Questions should be phrased to shed light, not only on suicidal tendencies, but also to reveal the young person's thoughts about methods and an appropriate time to commit the act. Wass stresses that this is important from a preventative perspective and for assessment of the seriousness of the situation. A young person who occasionally thinks or speaks of suicide, for example, is not quite the same as one who has considered issues, such as method, plans, motives etc. There is a need to explore the content and the intensity of young people's feelings. Do they have bad feelings occasionally, or do these constantly occupy their thoughts? Do they feel ashamed of having such feelings and ambivalent about their thoughts of suicide, or do they simply feel resigned and in a state of anticipation as to the orchestration of the deed? (ChildLine, *op cit*) Can they envisage a future? Have they considered turning to some of the professional support agencies that are available, and if so, do they want some direction and advice on how to obtain such help? It takes a great deal of skill, maturity and patience to work with depressed young people.

The greatest skill involves having true commitment to such practices, without becoming emotionally 'swamped' by them. Caring for people is hard, emotionally draining work.

There is also a need to change intolerant attitudes towards suicide and to promote the value and practice of 'good listening and talking' (Farmer, 1998). Much of the research so far has focused on young people who indicate a high suicide risk, but it is important to explore young people's attitudes and feelings towards suicide more generally. Research work has provided some interesting and useful results. Older adolescents appear to have a more negative attitude towards suicide than younger adolescents. This could be due to the fact that older young adults have considered the moral and ethical implications of suicide at a more complex level. Young women appear to have greater sympathy than young men (Wass, 1995). Research conducted by the Samaritans in 1998, suggests that young people tend to be less tolerant and understanding towards depression and suicide than older people. Fifty-seven percent of the younger people who took part in the study, considered that depressed people should 'pull themselves together', compared to 27% in the older group. A further question in the study aimed to explore perceptions of the level of stress in modern life. Again, there were differences between the older and younger group (69% of younger people agreed that life had become more stressful, compared to 82% in the older group), but these differences were more marginal.

The differences in response between the two questions are interesting. In comparisons between the two responses, it seems that younger people seem to be less sensitive to the link between stress and depression. The stronger feelings towards stress detected in the older group may reflect the realities of life. Most of the younger people who took part in this study had a sympathetic outlook on suicide:

> I suppose that everyone thinks about it at some time or another. In one way I think they are cowards. But in another way, you think 'well they must have felt really "gutted"'. I mean, there are time when you may think 'oh, I wish I was dead' but suicide is different. It's not the same feeling sick of life, and actually doing it. But, although I do think it's a shame when younger people do it, it's not as surprising as when an older person does it. I mean, the younger you are, the less understanding you have of the fact that you can cope. But an older person has already coped. So why not carry on coping?

The young person cited above emphasises that there are subjective dimensions contributing to suicide risk. He points out that although unhappiness is common to most people's experience, there are a variety of ways to make sense of, or rationalise such unhappiness. Techniques such as cognitive restructuring and cognitive behaviour therapy are two areas where professional support can be invaluable. The aim in this context is concerned with changing attitudes and the various ways that a person might view him/herself in relation to a given situation. From a health education and promotion perspective, behavioural change and self-empowerment approaches appear to be most compatible with such psychological therapies.

Behavioural change and self-empowerment approaches

Mackintosh (*op cit*) explains that the behavioural change approach aims to 'persuade the individual to adopt a particular lifestyle or listen to medical advice'. The self-empowerment approach aims to 'facilitate decision-making by improving how the individual feels about himself' so that 'by developing motivation, self-confidence and life skills the individual is in a better position to identify his own health needs and take actions to meet them'. The two approaches are similar insofar as they are based on individual perception and decision-making, and on developing self advocacy skills. The behavioural change model defines health from the point of view of the professional. Conversely, the empowerment model allows for diverse interpretations of health taken from vantage points defined and set by each individual client or patient. It appears that the more clinical psychological approaches 'fit in' better with the former approach, whereas the latter is more compatible with the more humanistic, counselling approaches.

Cognitive behaviour therapy provides a means for people to restructure their perceptions. This process of cognitive restructuring first encourages the person to identify persistent thoughts which are causing feelings of depression, then he/she can be encouraged to perceive such thoughts as 'distortions of reality that can be neutralised by challenging them rationally' (Wass, *op cit*). Various techniques, such as breathing exercises and distraction procedures can also be learned (Foy, 1992; Saigh, 1992). Additional behavioural strategies may involve physical exercise or monitoring of diet to help promote and maintain positive changes between therapy sessions. It is also common to combine such therapeutic approaches with drug therapies. Research suggests that combined drug and therapy approaches are most effective. Parents and educators can help young people to develop an immunity to the development of suicidal thoughts by teaching them specific techniques for dealing with painful life experiences. Stress reduction, cognitive restructuring and behavioural techniques are relatively easy to learn and, indeed, once learned, they are easy to teach (Wass, *op cit*). However, mistrust of health professionals was expressed quite explicitly by two of the participants.[4] They argued that this was due to the professional tendency to assign labels. Yet it seems that it is more what is implied in the terminology's use, rather than the use of labels in itself. The interviews, cited below, explored whether terms used in Erikson's framework could be substituted for medical terms, such as 'paranoia':

Christine: *You say that you found the psychologist unhelpful, why is that?*

Participant 1: Well she seemed to think that I should get over this idea that you need to be careful, I mean, this word paranoia, that really annoys me, it makes it seem that it's all your fault. When really, what my experience has taught me is that it isn't always wise to trust. If I hadn't been so trusting before (the trauma) then it would never have happened.

Christine: *Can we just discuss this word paranoia. Can I give you two examples? We could say, for the sake of argument, that either you are paranoid, or you have problems trusting people. Do you feel that there is any difference between these two ways of describing, well, what is if you like, the same thing?*

Participant 1: Yes, definitely, one is, well one is a label. It makes it seem like I am abnormal for responding, well as I see it, in a normal way. But, it is actually true to say that I do have difficulty trusting people. And I do see that, to the degree that I lack trust now, that is a problem, but it's a problem I can work with. Like, how can I put it. Paranoia, that suggests something inside you, something that was always there really. But when you say that a person has difficulty trusting people, yes, OK, it is the individual who has

4 We should also consider the difficulties faced by health care professionals, particularly those working in the field of mental health. For a more detailed and balanced discussion on this matter, see Sutherland (1998).

the problem... it's an individual who has a history if you see what I mean. And you can infer from that, that there may be something in that person's history that made them that way, something that wasn't my fault. So you are working with that. You know, you are still accepting that the person has a problem and that that person needs help or support to work with that problem. But at the same time you are not completely suggesting that it's all that person's fault.[5]

Participant 2: (responding to the same question) I think that is much better, to talk about trust and the lack of it, or whether or not, I mean, trust is something that varies and comes in degrees really isn't it? So it's not like a label that says, this is you, this is what you are like, for all time and in every situation. To say that a person has problems trusting people, that suggests that it's not all the time, you know. There are people they do trust and it's more true. You know, when you have had the experiences that I have had, you do take longer before you can trust people, and I think that is wise, although I'm also willing to admit that there are times when it might lead to problems. But even then, there's a sense of, it's not just my job to change, other people have a responsibility to do something, they have a responsibility to make trust possible. And that means behaving in a way that is decent, that will not erode trust. I think that is better because it recognises that people work with relationships, in all situations.

Christine: *If we take that further, say, instead of paranoia, lets work with lack of trust, instead of talking about interpersonal skills, lets talk about intimacy, isolation, despair. I mean, I'm kind of experimenting now, seeing what different words can mean.*

Participant 2: Definitely words like that are much better to work with, because they are human. You see, there is a tendency with all these medical labels, to make a

5 This participant who has suffered bouts of depression since she was the victim of an assault two years prior to the interview. Although admitting to depression, she did not volunteer any information as to whether or not she had ever experienced suicidal thoughts. This participant has had experience of seeing a psychologist and psychiatrist. She found both unhelpful.

> person seem less than human. If you see what I mean, most people are not paranoid, but you are. So you are part of a stigmatised group, you are different, less than human. Whereas, things like trust, isolation, intimacy, these are human, fully human. Every human being has problems with them, sort of, has to wrestle with them at some time or another. So it makes you a human being with a human problem. And I think that it would be good for professionals to recognise that, and to work with that. You see, this is how the professionals work with you, and to be honest, I think there is a bit of a power thing with a lot of professional people, especially in mental health. They might not think about it consciously, but they do think that you are less than human, like, it's their job to make you more human. And that is how they relate to you and it's a job. I mean, this active listening. It's a technique and to be honest, you can recognise it a mile off. It's a professional approach, it's based on like, they are told what to do. How to look at you, how to talk to you and I mean, even how and when to nod or shake their bloody heads. And, they are shaking and nodding their heads like this [imitates] and it's a technique they use to deal with people like you, people with a problem. But if you use language like that, it makes the whole thing human, and recognising that, they, including the professionals, have to work with you in a human way. You know, its not a medical or a health problem any more. It's a human problem.[6]

It appears then that adoption of some of Erikson's terms may offer useful and interesting possibilities for health care professionals. However, it would be inappropriate to end this discussion without expressing some regret at observing such mistrust of mental health care professionals. It cannot be denied that any association with mental health services can be stigmatising. It also has to be acknowledged that some mistrust is perhaps inevitable when we consider the reports of survivors of mental health services, who

6 This man developed a tendency towards becoming depressed in his early twenties. His story included various traumas and crises discussed during the interview, that had contributed to this.

have drawn our attention to issues, such as misuse of power and to the disabling effects of some therapies, ie. ECT (Beresford and Wallcraft, *op cit*). It is also important to note that counselling does not involve the medicalisation of experience and that it is often facilitating rather than oppressive (Rowan, 1983). Some very innovative approaches have developed within psychotherapy, such as art and drama therapy (Krystal, 1987; Early, 1993), and acknowledgement of their contribution to treatment cannot be stressed too highly. Counselling approaches are more concerned with working from the client's or patient's point of view and, as such, are more compatible with the empowerment rather than behavioural change approaches.

Encouraging young people to see the funny side of a situation is also helpful. Humour is a very effective method of stress reduction so it is worthwhile considering if we could develop child care strategies that help to promote happiness in young people (Wooten, 1998; Fanu, 1998). In recent years there has been an increase in research aimed at exploring the psychology of happiness (Argle, 1992). Myers and Diener (1996) write that:

> *Compared with misery, happiness is a relatively unexplored terrain for social scientists. Between 1967 and 1994, 46,380 articles indexed in Psychological Abstracts mentioned depression, 36,851 anxiety and 5,099 anger. Only 2,389 spoke of happiness, 2,340 life satisfaction and 405 joy.*

However scarce, recent research has identified four personality traits that appear to make people more predisposed to living happy lives (Argyle, 1992). These include the ability to like one's self (high self-esteem), the ability to feel in control of one's life (internal locus of control) optimism and extroversion. Involvement in relationships, community projects, meaningful activity and religious, spiritual pursuits also appear to improve people's potential for happiness. Intelligence and creativity are also important, although social context probably has the most influential impact on these variables. Montessori (1917) observed that people with high scores on each of these measures, possessed shrewd observation skills that enabled them to see the world with greater clarity than the average person. Over exposure to social and/or political injustice can tip the scales in a more negative direction, exposing such individuals to greater risk of depression. More recently Jamison (1996) has noted that 'recent studies indicate that a high number of established artists — far more than could be expected by chance — meet the diagnostic criteria for manic depression'. She also cautions that 'it would be wrong to label anyone who is unusually accomplished, energetic, intense, moody or eccentric as a manic depressive'.

We need to acknowledge the distinction between wit (which is often destructive because it involves ridicule) and humour, which, according to O'Connell (1995) is, 'the ability to avoid getting caught in mental ruts'. As noted, research into what happiness is and what causes it is relatively new. Making distinctions between wit and humour is difficult because of the contextual and relational qualities of both. What might be considered 'funny' in one context may be considered very offensive in another. Family members, spouses, or people involved in warm, close relationships, may consider it perfectly legitimate to make 'humorous' comments and observations that would be considered liberties if made by anyone else (Kenny, 1998a). If we relate this discussion to suicide prevention, there is much information available that aims to encourage depressed people to look for a 'funny' or 'light hearted' perspective to their situation. *Global Ideas Bank* (Arena, 1998; available on the Internet) provides a list of 45, mostly light-hearted reasons for 'saying no to suicide'. However, listed reasons, such as 'what if I die when I only meant to cry for help', may well have the opposite effect. First, it could be argued that the comment trivialises the distress experienced by many depressed, suicidal people. Second, it has the potential to make (some) suicidal people all the more determined to succeed, so that their attempt will not be seen as a 'cry for help' (*Chapter 2, p. 28*).

We also need to think very critically about encouraging oppressed groups to think differently about their situation. To adopt this approach rather than other alternatives (for example, enabling them to find means of challenging the situation by organising and placing pressure on authorities for change) might not necessarily be in that group's best interest. In such circumstances, such approaches may bring about short-term, temporary change. Should the source of unhappiness have a predominantly social as opposed to an individual basis, such an approach will reap few benefits in terms of long-term mental health. This is because it encourages the person to divorce him/herself from the realities of life. Bentall (cited by Fanu, 1998) argues that humour is grounded in irrational thinking. As such, it should be considered a pathology because it is 'statistically abnormal', reflects abnormal functioning and is associated with a lack of contact with reality. Health promotion includes some acknowledgement of the influence that social, political and economic structures can have on health. 'Bottom up' approaches, such as social change and community development advances are orientated to address inequalities in health caused by realities of poverty and related issues — unemployment, housing and the environment, eg. the neglect of inner cities.

Social change and community development approaches

Mackintosh (1996) explains that the goal underpinning the social change approach is to 'make healthy choices easy choices by changing the physical and social environment'. The focus of this approach is the environment and the political forces that have the power to bring about change. This perspective suggests that there are times when change is most quickly and effectively brought about by legislation (eg. no smoking policies). There is an emphasis on raising political awareness of the need for change, the organisation of groups and the development of strategies aimed at creating pressure for change. There are many social issues that contribute towards youth unhappiness and distress, including: unemployment, homelessness, isolation, and poverty. Priorities set by any one group working within the social change approach would depend on what the best perceived solution might be to a particular problem. The Citizens Income Study Centre, for example, operates on the premise that paying every citizen an adequate income, regardless of their individual circumstances, would be the most effective way to resolve poverty and all its related problems. This is argued on the assumption that the notion of 'jobs for all' will never become a reality. Other innovations might include the creation of social contexts that protect the unemployed from social isolation and loneliness by the creation of 'drop in' day centres and clubs for the unemployed (Breakwell, 1996), or campaigning for better quality, affordable and abundant housing for homeless young people.

Community development projects work from the perspective of the groups operating them. The aim is to 'help the group work together, find their common interests and fight their particular health cause'. Strategies may include enabling people to 'create self-help groups, facilitating the group and acting as a resource and supporter for the group' (Mackintosh, 1996). Relating this discussion to research, *Chapter 2* explored the issue of drug and substance abuse which can significantly increase a young person's risk of premature death and suicide. This is a cause of concern for many parents who may benefit from self-help groups designed to help them support their children.

Self-help groups are also useful for helping parents to develop the skills required to identify depression and provide appropriate support for their children. Being a parent is a rewarding but very challenging experience. If parents and their children are encountering problems, these problems can appear far more difficult and significant if the family group feel isolated. Self-help groups that enable parents and their children to work together to find solutions can reduce isolation, feelings of helplessness and create situations whereby information can be shared and skills developed.

The above discussion has been relatively brief, based on speculations of how some of the various approaches to health education and promotion might be utilised towards the promotion of mental health and the prevention of suicide. The aim has been to open up issues, to identify possible relationships and to make speculations for the future. The value of any programme can only be assessed by appropriate evaluation, and this takes time (Naidoo and Wills, 1994). What can be asserted with some confidence is that suicide, especially in the young, is a complex issue that demands recognition of both individual and collective responsibilities.

Young people should certainly be encouraged to share their frustrations with adults who are willing to listen and take such concerns seriously. But active listening on the part of parents is not always, in itself, enough. The young person may also need to be encouraged to explore the more positive options that are open to them. Young adults tend to prefer discussing their fears and concerns with their peers rather than their parents (Csikszentmihalyi and Larson, 1984). Under such circumstances, it can be very hard for a parent to know that anything is wrong. Some parents may feel overwhelmed at the prospect of discussing sensitive issues, such as death, or of opening up discussions that might enable them to recognise the existence of depression in their children. Even during adolescence when children are trying to develop some independence, the parents are still the most significant people in their lives. Attempts to discuss delicate issues can reap positive results, even if, initially, the parent meets with hostility. Sadly, some young people do become so unhappy that they commit suicide. This can happen despite any steps that may have been taken to prevent such an act. Alternatively, the suicide of a child might be the very first indication for the family that something was wrong. In the next chapter, we explore the impact of child suicide on survivors.

4

Survivors of suicide

Introduction

This chapter is concerned with the effects that the suicide of a child or young person can have on survivors; the emotional impact, the practicalities following the death and sources of support. Those who become bereaved due to suicide are referred to as 'survivors' (Wertheimer, 1991). She likens the emotional impact of suicide to that of a 'personal holocaust'. Wright (1993) considers it a triple burden; survivors have to cope with sudden death, the death of their child and the stigma of suicide. Each of these can be responsible for complicating the grieving process in different ways. There may be denial, a lack of ability to accept that a death has occurred, or to accept the accuracy of pertinent details connected with the loss (Kenny, 1998b; 1998c). Perhaps it is not surprising that symptoms expressed by many survivors are similar to those commonly associated with loss, but far more intense (Edmonds, 1990). The development of psychological autopsies in the 1960s, led indirectly to increased sensitivity to the needs of survivors. Interviews, initially conducted for the purpose of constructing a psychological profile of the deceased, revealed widespread intense, unresolved grief. Survivors had a deep need to talk of their grief, their loss and their own suicidal feelings. For many, the interviews proved cathartic, diminishing guilt and facilitating resolution of grief (Wertheimer, *op cit*).[1] Despite these findings, changes in attitudes and practice have been slow. In 1994 Rioch wrote:

> *Suicide of a child or adolescent, is one of the greatest tragedies and is likely to have a far-reaching effect, especially*

1 Similar findings have been reported by other researchers. Participants who took part in research on bereavement conducted by Hutchinson *et al* (1994), for example, thanked the researchers for having listened to them. Others, such as Coles (1989) and Kenny (1998c) felt that being given the opportunity to tell their stories acted as a form of catharsis. However, this does lead to ethical concerns (eg. is the researcher acting as a social enquirer, or a counsellor and, if so, should those who lack a counselling qualification be doing such research). This issue is explored extensively in a collection of papers published in Autumn 1998, *Oral History*, The Oral History Society, University of Essex.

on parents, other family members and the community. Much publicity is given locally, nationally and occasionally, internationally, to the young person following a suicide act; however, the anguish felt by the family does not appear to receive consideration.

It is hoped that this chapter will make a small contribution to an improved awareness of the impact of suicide.[2]

The emotional impact of suicide

A suicide in the family can place all its members at greater risk of becoming suicidal themselves. Severe trauma such as this can lead to 'cognitive constriction' (Leenaars,1995). This is a rigidity in thinking that narrows the individual's perceptive focus, leading to perceptual 'tunnel vision', causing distortions in emotions, logic and perception. Indirect expressions of this particular cognitive 'set' can include ambivalent, contradictory feelings, opinions and beliefs generally, or directed towards specific people. Conflicts emerge between wanting to survive and, at the same time, to escape unendurable pain.[3] Siblings of the dead child may consider suicide themselves, especially if silences and rifts in the family occur (The Compassionate Friends [TCF], 1993b). For such children, the feeling of isolation can be terrifying. For a few, suicide brings the dreadful possibility of following the dead brother or sister. If the pain gets too bad, 'I can always do what they did' (TCF, 1998b). One-parent families, with or without surviving children, can be very isolated and the grief of step-parents can be neglected or underestimated (TCF, 1998c).

If the cause of death was violent, this can be an even greater source of anxiety. A participant in this study commented that 'the method that they choose can be as significant as the fact that they did it'. She explains that violent death can make it appear to the bereaved, that the deceased had wished to punish them. Parents feel guilt because they were absent when the deceased needed them most

2 For readers interested in a recent comprehensive (and very readable) overview of how bereavement responses and practices differ across cultures, reference is made to the work of Parkes, Laungani and Young (1997) and their book *Death and Bereavement Across Cultures*, published by Routledge.

3 In such cases, Leenaars argues, the decision to attempt suicide may seem rather illogical and irrational because the driving force behind it, comes from the unconscious.

and because they were unable to prevent the act (TCF, 1993c). Survivors may torment themselves with concerns about whether or not the deceased suffered any pain. As one participant, speaking of a partner's suicide put it:

> Even now it comes over me, I think, I wonder if it hurt, you know? I like to think, well I hope that it was quick and that she was 'out of it' at the time that it happened. But there is always that nagging doubt, that 'I wonder if it hurt, I wonder if it hurt'. Even now I can find myself going over and over that in my mind. I can't bear to think that the very last thing felt was pain, you know? That she might even have changed her mind at the last minute, can you imagine the terror of that, to feel it coming on, to know it's too late. But I comfort myself by telling myself, well she planned it so carefully, she must have made the decision once and for all. But it's there, all the time, this nagging doubt. I expect it must be even worse in the event of a young person. I mean, an adult is responsible for themselves. But in the case of a young person, you always feel that as a parent, you are responsible. Yes, I must say, my heart really does go out to parents like that.

Parenthood is a lifelong commitment. A parent can feel responsible for their child's suicide no matter how old the child is. Many spend hours reading suicide books and literature hoping that this might provide some explanation, or clue to help them understand what had happened (Wertheimer, *op cit*). A participant in this study explained how, following the death of her son, she spent hours asking 'why, why, why?' She explained the first few months following his death[4]:

> It was terrible [sobs][5] no, no it's all right. It's just absolutely devastating to lose a child, even, I mean, it might seem strange to call an adult man of 24 a child. But he was, he is, he is my child, my little boy really. And of course it's the thing that they all say that you never expect that you are going to bury a child [voice breaks]. You expect that they will always be there, and of course, you just can't take it in. I mean, it was a nightmare, a complete nightmare for weeks and weeks afterwards. And for weeks you are wanting help, you feel desperate for someone to help you. But no one can. I mean, there can be dozens of people around you, but none of them can help, because they don't understand. You want company,

4 This participant's young adult son committed suicide.

5 At this point the participant began crying. The writer asked if the participant would like to discontinue the interview, but she gave her assurances that she would prefer to continue.

> and then when you get it, you want them to go. They irritate you, because they can't help, how can they help, how can they understand?

There is intense shock and disbelief and, as the participant above continues: 'life is full of "if onlys" you know? If only I'd done this; if only I'd have told him just how much I loved him when he was here; if only I'd noticed that something was wrong; and you know that you torment yourself with all these "if onlys".' Sudden death provides no opportunity to say 'goodbye'. Knowledge that the death has been brought about by a deliberate act generates a terrible source of guilt, as observed by the female medium who participated in the study:

> Guilt is one of the most difficult things, and I know you always get guilt when there is a bereavement. But in the case of a suicide, especially if it involves a young person, it is always far more severe. In my experience, guilt comes for all sorts of reasons. I mean, knowledge that they [the survivors] couldn't accept them for what they were; guilt that maybe you could have prevented it; that maybe there were signs that you missed. One young woman who came to see me, her son had committed suicide and she was a one-parent family, you know? So there was guilt there, that maybe if she'd have been a better mother, maybe if she hadn't gone to work, maybe if she'd not been so busy. But, when someone dies, we always think of the things that we could have done, that we should have done. The thing is, we are human, we make mistakes. Or we may have responsibilities that make it hard for us to be perfect, we can only do our best. But the guilt is one of the worst things in my experience.

The grief of associates of the deceased, whose relationship with him or her had been secret, for example, in the case of gay or extra marital relationships, can be intense. This is a grief that cannot be openly acknowledged (Wertheimer, *op cit*). Below, an older woman recalls her experience of losing a lover:

> I was in the position that I couldn't share my grief with anyone. I had to get on with my life, but I did have very deep periods of melancholy. I got rid of every single thing that he owned, apart from a tie. I kept that for ten years. I just felt that I had to keep something, and, I kept it very well hidden and every now and again I'd take it out and look at it; his blue tie, he wore that more than anything else that he wore... when I finally got rid of that, it was the last physical act, the last act to say that I had and I could let go.

Suicide notes rarely provide the answer to what led to the suicide. Some contain messages telling survivors not to blame themselves, others explicitly allocate blame. The participant above further commented on the suicide note left to her, that had a perceived subtext reading 'see what you have done to me'. Such experiences can have a terrible effect on survivors, who can feel that they have effectively murdered the victim. This participant commented that she felt guilty and angry at the same time when she read the letter. Her anger stemmed from her belief that it was he (the lover) not she who had been responsible for the death. No matter what the content of a suicide note, survivors when reading them have some sense of the victim's helplessness at the time that they committed the act. This can be very distressing. The coroner or police may withhold notes when direct blame is evident, although this, too, can be damaging. There are times when what is imagined can be far worse than the reality (Wertheimer, *op cit*).

Individuals have their own, unique way of grieving. Sometimes this can lead to misunderstandings and resentment. Men may find it difficult to express their emotions and, indeed, may be expected to return to work and carry on as normal a short time after the death. Sometimes the prospect of returning to work can be even more difficult if the individual works in a professional capacity. They may be accustomed to dealing with bereavement and suicide. The spouse of one participant was a caring professional and assumed after his son's suicide, that his colleagues might be judgemental, critical of his (apparent failure) to prevent the suicide. The man's fears were unfounded and he found that his colleagues were 'wonderful' (to use the terminology of his spouse), doing all that they could to help and support him. 'The family may become united in their grief, or the suicide may lead to the break up of the family.' However, when this happens Wrobeski (1991) suggests that disharmony may have existed prior to the suicide.[6] In addition to their own sense of loss, grandparents witness their children grieving (TCF, 1993a). Consumed by their grief, parents often prove inadequate sources of support for surviving children (TCF, 1993b). This was noted by one of the funeral directors who took part in this study:

> The thing that really upsets you is the death of a child, especially if it has been caused by a suicide. It's not so much dealing with the body, it's the funeral really, and more than anything, it's the effects that it has on the kids. I mean, usually

6 Rioch, *op cit*.

> if kids go to a funeral, in my experience, the adults are pretty good, but not when there's a suicide, more often than not I mean. I've been to funerals where, I'd say quite a lot of the kids are stood on their own, the adults, they are all talking amongst themselves. And they can't seem to see how upset the kids are. And it upsets you, it really does, because it's almost as if the impact has been so great on them [the adults] that they have lost the ability to see what it has done to anyone else, especially the kids. And you really feel that you want to intervene, to go over and say 'I'm sorry about your friend' I mean, if it's a kid of their own age, it really does hit them hard. I don't think that they mean to be insensitive, I think that they are just too full of their own grief really, to see the children. It's as if they are not there, they just don't seem able to see them.

Brothers and sisters of the deceased may feel that they are to blame, especially if they had an argument with the deceased prior to the death (Lake, 1984). TCF (1998b) acknowledge how difficult it can be to explain to young children what has happened. Children, as discussed in *Chapter 1*, have an immature understanding of death to begin with, but it can be almost impossible for them to understand something as complicated as suicide. In such situations, parents have the added burden of their own grief. This can complicate their ability to explain anything to anyone, least of all children. However, despite these difficulties, TCF recommend that some honesty and openness are necessary. Although it may be impossible for a young child to comprehend what has happened, the parents should try to explain things as clearly as possible. It is also important to check that there is consistency in the stories that different people are telling the child. TCF note that explanations need to be ongoing and revisited over the years. As the child's intellectual abilities change, explanations need to be adjusted to 'fit' his/her ability to understand. Finally, TCF note the importance of making surviving siblings feel loved and secure. Observing these recommendations requires great skill and sensitivity. This can be very difficult when parents are in an extreme state of grief themselves, but without such reassurance, the child may feel rejected. Feelings of rejection are common in cases of suicide, and may hit the family member or friend who finds the body harder. Initial reactions to the death will 'vary from that of shock, numbness and disbelief to open expressions of emotions and hysterical screaming' (Rioch *op cit*).[7] The parents may be overwhelmed by the

7 Rioch (*op cit*) asserts that parents should be given a private room in which they can express their emotions.

finality of the situation. One of the funeral directors interviewed observed an abrupt change in parents as this reality 'hits home'. He explained that there is, at first, numbness, then it 'hits them like a sledgehammer'. Many years of experience had failed to provide him or his colleagues with emotional immunity to such experiences.

What about children of people who commit suicide? The loss of a parent in childhood can contribute to mental health problems, such as schizophrenia in later life (Watt and Nicholi, 1979). Young people are amazingly resilient and with adequate support from surviving parents or other caretakers, they can adjust to the loss. The psychiatric adjustment of surviving adults is very important (Kranzler, 1990). A child's security becomes threatened by the death of a caretaker, whereas loss of a sibling or peer brings home his/her own mortality. The bereaved child may feel anger and guilt at the fact that he/she has survived, especially if caretakers compare the surviving child unfavourably with the one who has died. The person finding the body will be in an intense state of shock. In the case of an adolescent or young adult, this might not be a relative or even a friend. A participant interviewed for this study, commented on the tragedy of young people, who die alone. In 'bed-sit land' the presence of an unpleasant smell might be the first indication that something is wrong. The condition of the body and of the room may increase the sense of shock.[8] Another participant commented on the effect this can have on a younger person:

> For those who find the body, oh that is a shock, especially if it's a young person, and especially if the young person who finds them had spent some time with them before. Because they will torment themselves, looking for hints or suggestions. And they can have some terrible, terrible nightmares. One young woman who came here, her friend hung himself, she found him. And do you know? For months and months, she couldn't close her eyes, without this image of him hanging there, coming back. She became really very desperate, because she believed that it was all she was ever going to see. She kept saying 'when will it go away, how will I ever take that image

8 This participant was a funeral director. He explained how a corpse can decompose very quickly after death, particularly if the room is hot and if the death involved the use of drink or drugs, which cause discolouration. The main cause of sorrow (and according to this participant, professionals who deal with the practical aspects of death often encounter experiences that cause them great sorrow) was the knowledge that the deceased had died alone and in a state of despair. The participant further reported that he and many of his colleagues never really developed emotional immunity to such deaths.

away' ... it can have a very strong impact on them. In this case, luckily this young woman did go for help. And with help it did eventually go away, this image. But I know of another one, well she ended up having to go for help, or rather, well, in this case she had a nervous breakdown. She was tormented, tormented by this image. In this case it was a group of friends. They were all living in the same group of flats, and they like, sort of used to look out for each other. But this particular night, one of them, a young girl, she went to bed early, or so she said. And this other one [the friend who found the deceased] found her in bed. She'd been there a while, I think she had taken tablets, taken an overdose. Well from all accounts, it wasn't a pretty sight... it was a terrible, terrible shock to her. She was only a young girl, to suffer a terrible shock like that. Her parents I believe [of the deceased] were very good. They even offered to pay I believe for this young woman who found her to get therapy. She refused, or so I'm told. But she needed it in the end... because like I say, she had a breakdown.[9]

However, responses to suicide are not always as dramatic (or indeed negative) as we might assume (Wertheimer, *op cit*). If the deceased has made many attempts in the past, there may actually be some relief from the pressure and continuous anticipation that a suicide might happen. In cases such as the second discussed above, the parents appear to have resigned themselves to such a possibility. Wrobeski (1991) comments that, 'although life can never be the same again for a family following a suicide, life has to go on' and that 'it can sometimes be helpful to consider the fact that, the worse that can happen already has'.[10] A similar point was made by a participant whose friend (a heroin addict) died of an accidental drug overdose. Speaking of a conversation with the mother of the deceased he recalls:

Well his mother, she was in a terrible state, as you can imagine, but in a sad kind of way, she had a kind of acceptance about her, it was difficult to explain. But she did say when I spoke to her, you know, I went over to ask her how she was. And she said, 'well, I'm upset, but to be honest, not that shocked because I knew he would do it eventually. I mean, playing with fire like that, and we did all we could... ' and all this. And she did say that in a way, she had already lost her son a long time ago, which I suppose is true. I mean, they do

9 Participant aged about 60–65 years of age. This participant has had much experience of supporting people who have been bereaved, especially due to a suicide.

10 Cited by Rioch, 1994, p. 35.

> change and like, what kind of future can you see? I mean, I have no kids myself, but I'd imagine that you have some kind of future in mind, but with drugs, all that is taken away, anyway.[11]

The participant above refers to two phenomena; those of 'anticipatory grieving', and 'social death'. Each can be initiated before biological death occurs. Both are most commonly observed when the likelihood of a death appears strong.[12] It is commonly asserted that, due to reduced mortality in the young, the death of a child carries an added burden.[13] There is an assumption that parents in particular will have greater difficulty accepting the death of a child. Kenny argues that, due to a variety of issues in the last few years, such as AIDS, rising suicide rates and drug addiction, this assumption needs to be revised. The expectation that parents will outlive their children is not universal and is becoming increasingly vulnerable.[14] This is a view that some parents have expressed to Kenny in the course of her research. Some of these parents have young adult children known to be experimenting with drugs. Such parents feel desperate, helpless and unsure of how to protect their children. There is anger about the lack of access to information, information that is not very helpful and the lack of support for bereaved parents. Sometimes, the stress of parent/ child conflict during adolescence causes the latter to leave home.

Despite the potential isolation caused by living alone, some young people organise themselves into informal community support systems.[15] This can be helpful, but it does not always offer protection against depression or suicide. When a suicide does occur in such circumstances, the effects can be devastating. For members of 'outsider' groups, those who lack confidence, and those who live 'on the margins', suicide of a peer can challenge belief that survivors had it in their ability to be, at least, a good friend. No one, parents, siblings or peers may know what caused the suicide. The opportunity to ask the young person how he/she feels has gone. The child is dead. Paralysed by shock, hopelessness and confusion, parents find it

11 24-year-old male participant.

12 The author discusses each of these concepts in greater depth in *A Thanatology of War* (1998), Quay Books, Mark Allen Publishing Ltd.

13 This is frequently contrasted with the reactions of previous generations, when, due to high mortality rates in the young, people were assumed to be more accepting of child deaths.

14 Kenny notes that not all the people who have expressed this opinion have agreed to be interviewed, or to fill in questionnaires. Although very reluctant to formally take part in her research, such people have, at her request, agreed to her referring to the matter in this publication.

15 This was observed by a female participant speaking of 'bed-sit' land in Bolton.

difficult even to decide how to dispose of their child's body (TCF, 1993c).

Dealing with the practicalities following a suicide

No matter how painful, practicalities have to be dealt with. In the event of a suicide, one of the first ordeals facing the parents will be the formal identification of the body. A bereaved mother remarked during her interview, that she was unable to recognise her son. She was convinced that a mistake had been made. His hair was arranged in a style that (she noted with considerable irritation) did not suit him.[16] With care and skill, unsightly and disfiguring parts can be disguised, even when the body is badly mutilated. This makes the identification procedure less traumatic. Each family member should be encouraged to make independent decisions about viewing the body before it is taken to the undertaker's premises (Rioch, *op cit*). During his interview, a funeral director challenged the assumption that it is always beneficial to view the body. Responses to viewing the body can be extreme if it is mutilated or decomposed. In such cases, he considered it the responsibility of the funeral director to point out that viewing might not be advisable.

If the bereaved decide against viewing the dead person immediately, they should be informed that further opportunities will be provided at the undertaker's premises. Parents may wish to participate in preparing the body for the funeral. Others may find consideration of such practicalities intolerable (Rioch, *op cit*). One of the funeral directors said that asking about the disposal of the body can be one of the hardest questions because this brings home the reality of the death. Parents will be informed that an inquest is necessary to establish the cause of death. It may be some months after the death before the family receive news of the verdict. This may prove an additional source of distress, particularly if the conclusions are at odds with the family's perception of what happened. An 'open verdict' may be recorded in the absence of a suicide note. This may be comforting, but not always. No matter how painful, some families prefer honesty and a clear explanation of what

16 This mother's son had died in early adolescence. This was an accidental death, not a suicide. She agreed to be interviewed informally, and to some of the information she provided being used for this book. However, she would not agree to a taped interview.

has happened rather than vagueness and ambiguity (TFC, 1998b). The inquest may be very difficult, especially if it attracts press reporters who add to the distress by publishing sensational reports. Bolton (1987, cited by Rioch) advocates pro active steps to minimise press reporting and suggests that a friend or family member writes an account for the press. Rioch (1994) notes that, 'the attitude of neighbours who may imply blame can contribute to the parent's feelings of guilt, and in addition, any hostility from relatives can intensify these feelings'.

Participants in this study commented on the distressing effects of press reports.[17] One spoke of her experience when a young man committed suicide after she terminated her relationship with him. Her perception that the newspaper reports of the incident implied blame on her part, was very distressing and, she believed, encouraged discrimination and a judgemental attitude from her peers. She commented:

> It's amazing how all sorts of people think that they have the right to speak, you know, to put in their 'halfpenny's worth'. And stories like that do not help, people read the paper, and think that they know the whole story. It really was a terrible thing. I mean, it brought shame and embarrassment on the whole family, and you know, quite a few members of my family, they wouldn't allow me in the house for a long time after. I found it very hard to go out for a long time, and I became very depressed. I felt that the whole world blamed me. But there was more to it than that [report in the paper] I mean, he had lots of other problems, but none of those were mentioned. It really was a very, very difficult time in my life and, what made it worse was, I blamed myself. Even though I knew it wasn't my fault, I blamed myself, so that kind of thing did not help. I would say that, of all the grieving that I have done in my life that [the suicide] was the hardest. That's the biggest and the hardest of all the grieving that I have done, and it wasn't helped by those newspaper reports, not at all.

Newspaper reports on suicide are diverse. More space is devoted to stories that report deaths of young people. Survivors can find the presence of the press and the subsequent reports very distressing.

17 These participants included, a mother whose son had committed suicide, a woman who experienced a suicide when a young man she had been involved with, committed suicide (this happened many years ago, before the woman had married) and a man whose wife committed suicide. Ages were not provided by any of the participants, but all were above retirement age.

They may fear that unfair moral judgements will be made. Survivors resent the intrusion and having the details of their private lives publicly reported in the local papers. A survivor in this study felt so grieved by the reports of his partner's suicide that he 'never forgave them' (the reporters) and 'never, bought the local paper again'. He also objected to having his private life published. He felt very aggrieved that the press had not consulted him on what was to be reported. This participant recalled that his son had great difficulty fitting in at school. The knowledge that his school friends, and their parents, had read the reports caused the boy great embarrassment. His father empathised with this because he also avoided friends and neighbours for many months afterwards. This father explained that whenever he read of a suicide, the pain and grief of his own experience came back to him and that 'my heart really goes out to these people, because I think, reading this, how must they feel. As if they haven't been through enough'.

Another survivor of suicide described the anger and resentment she felt at seeing reporters write down details of her son's death during the inquest. She approached one reporter and asked, 'have you got what you want now?' at which the latter replied, 'it's my job'. While acknowledging this, the participant was hurt by the coldness of response and the fact that 'the newspaper reports were very hurtful'. In this case the press had adopted a sympathetic approach. But the participant felt that this presented her son in a negative light. Following the reports, a friend of this mother had described the son's suicide as an act of selfishness, to which the former responded 'but he wasn't selfish, and I didn't want people to think of him like that. I didn't want people to think about what might have been bad about him. I wanted him to be remembered for the good he had done'.

Another survivor said that reports of her nephew's suicide were not as bad as she had expected them to be. This was because sensationalism was reduced to a minimum.[18] This participant also gained some comfort from the fact that the reporters had presented a very positive assessment of her nephew's personality. Sometimes reports can be helpful to the bereaved. Positive and sympathetic reports can help to raise awareness about the needs of the bereaved. Although press reports of a suicide cannot be avoided, there are ways to reduce their traumatic effects. TCF (1998b) recommend that parents release a brief statement to the press, along with a photograph of the

18 Female participant, interviewed concerning her nephew who committed suicide.

child. This can make the press more responsive to requests that the family's privacy be respected. The humiliation of having private grief publicly reported can be intensified in families where communication is poor and the suicide is not openly discussed. Press reports deny survivors the opportunity to tell the details in their own time and in their own way. Inaccurate reports increase distress (Wertheimer, *op cit*).

The expense of the funeral can add further to the distress of the parents. It is important to give them information, in writing, of the availability of grants. Funerals can be a great source of comfort (Fulton, 1995). They provide an opportunity for people to talk and, in doing this, allocate some meaning to the death. In the case of a suicide the family may prefer gathering together a few close friends and family members to share in the proceedings. The service may include some acknowledgement of the fact that suicide caused the death. Demonstrations of acceptance such as this can be very helpful (Wertheimer, *op cit*). Local ministers provide valuable and experienced sources of advice and comfort. They can be of great assistance to parents who are having to plan their child's funeral. The 'funeral may help provide great comfort and a lasting happy memory' (Rioch, 1994). However, some funerals can be counterproductive. Sometimes, family arguments about who is to blame for the suicide can erupt. Some people might be excluded altogether. Wertheimer notes that, 'regardless of whether or not the bereaved have any religious sentiments themselves, they can still be very distressed by fears that the deceased might be dammed to eternal hell' and that 'many survivors want some assurance that that the deceased will not be punished'. She continues, 'although suicide victims are no longer denied a proper funeral service and burial, suicide and religion often remain uneasy bedfellows.'

Support for the bereaved

The suicide of a young person will have an impact on the whole community. To ensure a quick and appropriate response Rosenberg *et al* (1989) recommend the implementation of similar strategies to those mobilised due to incident plans.[19] The advantage of local action plans is that they assist carers and prevent outbreaks of panic.

19 Major incident plans are planned strategies that can be mobilised in any locality in response to a major incident.

They also facilitate 'an effective response to the needs of other children in the locality, who will be confused and upset at the death of a friend' (Rioch, 1994). Rioch advocates professional, multi-disciplinary involvement from professionals, skilled in the provision of emotional and psychological support, who can advise on the official details. The head teacher of the dead child's school will be the first of such professionals to receive news of the death. The local action plan advocated by Rioch is envisaged to 'support staff and pupils when they hear of the tragic death of their young friend'. She also notes that 'teaching staff should anticipate that the death may have an adverse effect on the school performance of brothers and sisters of the young person'. Two of the participants commented on the effect that the suicide had on the school performance of surviving siblings. A bereaved mother provided insight into the effect such trauma can have on a person's intellectual ability:[20]

> In the first few months my biggest problem was getting up in the morning. I would just lie there, and even though I was awake and not tired even, I just could not move, just couldn't motivate myself. Then, as time when on, I'd try to keep myself busy, but I found that my concentration had just gone, I just could not concentrate on anything, not even writing up a shopping list. I was really forgetful, and when people were talking to me, I just wasn't there, I was like, nodding, as if I was listening, but nothing was sinking in. The problem was, I didn't want to listen to other people, if you know what I mean, I wanted them to listen to me. Even now, I can find myself drifting off... it really did affect my concentration very badly.

Following the suicide of a child, the bereaved family will come into contact with a variety of professional people. The attitude and skills of professionals is crucial. The survivors who took part in this study spoke of the need to talk about their grief. This chapter concludes with a discussion of the kind of formal and informal support that may be available, drawn mainly from the work of Wertheimer (*op cit*). She found the ease with which the bereaved gain access to support systems varies depending on matters, such as availability, how well publicised these are and whether or not effective referral services

20 The writer acknowledges that responses might differ in a child. There were no young children interviewed for this study, due to ethical considerations. However, the information is useful, because it provides some insight (though in the case of children, this is tentative) into how, for example, school activities such as reading, comprehension, indeed the ability to learn, problem solve or take in new information could adversely affect school performance.

exist. Sometimes, the family had stumbled on such services in a rather haphazard fashion.

The friend of a bereaved mother reported that she was very bitter because she received no support when her 17-year-old son died from a drug overdose.[21,22] Most people have a general practitioner. Some of the participants in Wertheimer's study reported that their GPs had been very unhelpful.[23] The prescription of tablets appeared insensitive, especially if overdose had been the cause of death. However, GPs are also human and vulnerable. They may be aware of their lack of skill and knowledge and feel very inadequate and guilty. There are considerable variations in availability of services, such as counselling or psychotherapy. Advice, counselling and support services for the bereaved are becoming more common in Britain, but are found mainly in more densely populated areas. Access to services in London, for example, is very good, as it tends to be in other large towns and cities. There is usually less accessibility in the more rural areas.[24,25]

Other survivors of suicide include professional people. In recent years there has been an increased sensitivity to people, such as train drivers. Such individuals can now claim compensation under the Criminal Injuries Compensation Scheme because of the profound impact such experiences can have on them. Many have long lasting problems after the event, such as insomnia, recurrent nightmares, heightened stress and anxiety (Finney, 1988). The two funeral directors, who took part in this study, spoke at length of the

21 In this case an 'open verdict' had been recorded because the young man had been a heroin addict. It was not clear whether the death had been accidental.

22 Much seems to depend on the goodwill and commitment of individual professionals. The author has interviewed two health care professionals, both working in a local hospital, who have prepared information leaflets for bereaved relatives. A much larger scale study would be required to identify how formal and common such practice is.

23 However, it is important to note that more and more GPs now offer a counselling service.

24 TCF (1998b) note that the best people to approach in order to gain access or information to services such as this, include doctors, religious leaders and local social services. The author notes that the local health or education service may also be useful. The next chapter provides a list of organisations.

25 Only one participant who took part managed to gain access to formal support, ie. was informed of TCF by a friend. Four others gained support, not from a counsellor but from a medium who gave them advice about local professional counselling. This person acted as a source of information as well as a medium. While recognising that this study had a much smaller sample size, this may indicate that attention needs to be drawn to issues, such as level of education, locality and social class. We also need to take into account that most of the survivors of suicide had experienced their loss, on average, five years or more before the interview.

emotional impact that a suicide can have on them. Handling mutilated or decomposed bodies are further sources of stress, as are experiencing the grief of relatives and observing bereaved siblings. The interviews provided by these participants were very contradictory. On the one hand they insisted that they were able to 'switch off', on the other, they admitted to having occasional nightmares.

For some, informal support groups are preferred to more professional sources of support.[26] Most of the participants in this study preferred to attend the local Spiritualist Church, and some had visited a medium.[27] This was partly due to an expressed need to make contact with the dead child, to gain some assurances that he or she was safe. One participant explained how in the case of a child 'you want to know that they go on somehow, that they have not come to an end'. Three of the participants also challenged the view that the bereaved should learn to 'let go' of the dead person. Two admitted to regular feelings that the dead person was present in the room, to sometimes talking to him or her.[28] One of the mediums who participated in the study is cited below:

> Most of the people who come to see me want to know more or less the same things, but you can find out for sure just by questioning them in the beginning. For a start, especially with a young person, with suicide there is a terrible sense of guilt and blame. They want someone to take that away. They want a message from their loved one, telling them that they are not to blame, not to be guilty — they need to be told that quite clearly and sometimes more than once. Secondly, they want to know that their loved one is safe and that they are happy and at peace. Now sometimes they [the bereaved] get frustrated, because they don't get at first the person that they want, it might be another dead relative, an older person most usually. But the message, if they are patient, will come through that other person. You see love, when we move on to that other state of development, we take a lot of our feelings, like shame and guilt with us. If the person feels ashamed of what they did, they may hide, they often do in fact, until they know for sure that those they left behind are not angry with them.

26 Anger and resentment in such cases might not be directed solely towards health care professionals. The bereaved mother discussed in this study, apparently blamed the school that her son attended. Her perception was that, had the boy not been excluded, he might not have become dependent on drugs in the first place.

27 Two mediums, one male and one female, took part in this study. The female medium is cited above.

28 This need for the bereaved to maintain some relationship with the dead has also been noted by Weinstein, 1998. See reference list for details of his paper.

> When they are hiding like that, they need another person to make that contact.

Faith in science, religion and the paranormal was once considered incompatible. Religion represented mere ignorance and superstition, whereas science offered incontestable facts — a feature of the enlightenment (Bradshaw, 1996). One feature of post-modernism has been a challenge to the authority of science. The distinction between science and religion is becoming increasingly blurred. More and more people who might formally have died are now being 'revived'. An astonishing number of 'near death' experiences have been reported in recent years (Bailey and Yates, 1996). This suggests that we should, perhaps, be less dismissive than we might once have been of accounts, such as that given by the medium cited above.[29] Beliefs in the paranormal should never be dismissed. However, this text offers insufficient space to do justice to a discussion of the issue. It is sufficient to open up thoughts and possibly debate on the subject, given that spiritualism was a very strong theme to emerge in this research. When asked about professional support, participants appeared reluctant to discuss this, and there appeared to be a suspicion of more professional sources of support.[30] The cost was also important: when asked about professional help such as counselling, three participants commented that few unemployed or working-class people can afford private counselling.

Bereavement support groups can be very helpful. Only one participant in this study attended meetings of the local survivors of suicide (SOS) an associate group of The Compassionate Friends (TCF). However she found these meetings extremely helpful. TCF was founded by the Reverend Simon Stephens in 1969. Membership of TCF is open to all bereaved parents, grandparents and siblings. Associate membership is available to relatives and friends of the bereaved and professionals who have an interest in bereavement. Group support and contact are available at meetings, in letters, telephone calls, indeed, any form of communication that is available

29 Many such survivors report that the experience has virtually changed their lives and priorities, many losing a concern for material possessions and gaining satisfaction, instead, from experiencing the more spiritual aspects of life. Most also report having no fears of death, whatsoever.

30 This is Kenny's perception and it is caused by the lack of willingness of most of her participants to discuss professional support. It might also be possible that participants received support, such as professional counselling, but were unwilling to admit to this. It is regrettable to have to acknowledge that, in some communities, there remains a stigma attached to professional counselling.

to suit the needs and characteristics of a particular bereavement group. The TCF also has a list of books, leaflets and fact sheets that provide information about different forms of bereavement, and a postal library. Associate groups exist (eg. SOS) to support bereaved people with specific needs due to the nature of their loss (TCF, 1998a). Further information about TCF and other support services is provided in the *Appendix*. We should not conclude this discussion without taking into account the value of family and friends. One of the participants in this study reported that her friends had been very supportive. The most comforting thing for her was that they had been willing to listen when she spoke of her son.[31] The participant emphasised that provision of the opportunity to talk was important, even if the friends made no comment throughout the discussion. Lukas and Seiden (1987) state that 'good listening permits good talking'. Support is essential in helping people cope with any bereavement, but such support is especially important in the case of a suicide.

Families may seem the most obvious source of support. Wertheimer noted that help and support are often available from friends and family immediately after a death, but this is gradually withdrawn. After a few weeks, the initial numbness and shock wear off, leaving the bereaved acutely aware of their pain. In addition, there are times when, no matter how close the family happens to be, people want to talk to someone who is uninvolved. Sometimes this 'outside person' can be a good friend, but at other times the bereaved person may prefer to use a professional service, or a support group. Wertheimer suggests that the combined support of friends and professional services can be extremely effective.

Conclusion

This chapter has explored the emotional impact that the suicide of a child can have on survivors. Survivors have included the family — parents, grandparents and siblings — peers and professional people. Difficulties can be increased by practicalities, such as having to identify the body, the coroner's report and the funeral. Outside influences, such as newspaper reports and the attitude of people who

31 The friends this participant referred to, appear to have been very empathetic indeed. She reported that they were willing to stop and listen to her talk about her son, even in public places and, indeed, even when on some occasions, she broke down in tears.

come into contact with the bereaved can also complicate or ease the trauma. Finally, the importance of support and the various sources available have been discussed. The *Appendix* lists some of the support organisations available.

Appendix

Organisations and bereavement support services

This information is taken from leaflets produced by the following organisations and CRISIS. Most of the listed organisations provide a range of services, such as telephone help lines and advice lines, letter and e-mail communication services and local support groups. They also provide information about the availability of local professional services, such as counsellors and psychotherapists.

Young minds:
102–108 Clerkenwell Road, London, ECIM 5SA
Tel: 0207 336 8445

The Samaritans:
10, The Grove, Slough, Berkshire, SL1 1QP
Tel: 01753 532713

MIND (largest national mental health organisation)
Granta House, 15–19 Broadway, London, E15 4BQ
Tel: 0208 519 2122

See also groups associated with MIND, including:

Diverse Minds (concerned with the delivery of mental health services that are appropriate to the needs of ethnic minority groups): Tel: 0208 519 2122

Rural Minds (concerned with the promotion of mental health and health services for people who live in rural areas)
Tel: 0247 41 43666

MINDLINK (advice network supported by and for support of survivors of mental health services) Tel: 0208 519 2122

Hackney MIND (residential provision): Whiston Housing Project, 38 Whiston Road, London E2 8BW
Tel: 0207 913 5326

CRISIS (provides support, housing, food and clothing for homeless people): First Floor, Challenger House, 42 Adler Street, London E1 1EE
Tel: 0207 655 8300

Support for people bereaved due to a suicide

The Compassionate Friends
53 North Street, Bristol BS3 1EN
Tel: 0117 966 5202; Help line: 0117 953 9639

Also has associate groups for:

Survivors of suicide (SOS)

Bereaved grandparents

National Association of Bereavement Services
Second Floor, 4 Pinchin Street, London E1 1SA
Admin/Fax: 0207 709 0505; Help line: 0207 709 9090

CRUSE
Headquarters at: 126 Sheen Road, Richmond, Surrey TW9 LUR
Tel : 0208 940 4818 (for details of the nearest group to check on their training programme)

London Association of Bereavement Services
Tel: 0207 700 8134 (answer phone). Some of the bereavement services affiliated to the London Regional Office of National Association of Bereavement Services run training courses and study days which are available to both members and non-members
www.bereavement.org.uk

Cancer link
Now run a training programme. Details from: 0207 833 2818. Venues throughout the UK

Other avenues

Local Citizens' Advice Bureau

Local Adult Education Centre

Local Establishments of Higher Education

Local libraries

Health clinics and GP practices

References

Abramson LY, Seligman MEP, Teasdale JD (1978) Learned helplessness in humans: critique and reformulation. *J Abnorm Psychol* **87**: 49–74

Ainsworth MDS, Wittig BA (1969) Attachment and exploratory behaviour of one year olds in a strange situation. In: Foss BM, ed *Determinants of Infant Behaviour*, Vol. 4. Methuen, London

Akenhurst R, Godfrey C, Hulton J, Robertson E (1991) *The Health of the Nation: An Economic Perspective on Target Setting*. Centre of Health Economics, University of York, York

Aldridge D (1998) *Suicide: The Tragedy of Hopelessness*. Jessica Kingsley, Bristol

American Psychiatric Press (1998)*Teen Suicide*. Public information fact sheet, Internet publication: http://www.appi.org; e-mail: mrscott@aacap.org

Anthony S (1971) *The Discovery of Death in Childhood and After*. Penguin Press, USA

Arena J (1998) *Arena's Emotional MASH tent: Front-line Encouragement including 45 personally tested reasons to say 'no' to suicide*. e-mail: Jarena@tcccom.net

Argle M (1992) *The Social Psychology of Everyday Life*. Routledge, London

Aries P (1960) *Centuries of Childhood: A Social History of Family Life*. Baldick R, trans. Knoff, New York

Atkinson JM (1975) *Discovering Suicide: Studies in the Social Organization of Sudden Death*. International Self-Counselling Press Ltd, Canada

Bailey LW, Yates J (1996) *The Near Death Experience*. Routledge, London

Balkwin H (1972) Depression: A mood disorder in children and adolescents. *MD State Med J* **21**(6): 55–61

Bandura A, Ross D, Ross S (1961) Transmission of aggression through imitation of aggressive models. *J Abnorm Soc Psychol* **63**: 575–82

Bandura A (1977) *Social Learning Theory*. Prentice Hall, Englewood Cliffs, USA

Bandura A (1980) The stormy decade: fact or fiction? In: Muss RE, ed. *Adolescent Behavior and Society: A Book of Readings*. 3rd edn. Nardon *House, New York*

Bandura A (1982) Self-efficacy mechanism in human agency. *Am Psychol* **37**: 122–47

Barraclough B (1986) The relationship between mental illness, physical illness and suicide. In Morgan J, ed. *Suicide: Helping Those at Risk*. Kings College, London

Baric L (1985) The meaning of words: health promotion. *J Inst Health Educ* **23** (1): 367–72 (cited by Mackintosh, 1996)

Barnes C, Mercer C, eds (1996) *Exploring the Divide: Illness and Disability*. The Disability Press, University of Leeds, Leeds

Baume P (1996) *Suicide in Young People*. Australian Institute for Suicide Research and Prevention, Internet Fact sheet: http://www.gu.edu.au/gwis/airsrap/htm

BBC1 (1998) *Inside Story: Fallen Hero: The Story of Justin Fastenu* (Thursday, 3 September)

Beresford P, Wallcraft J (1997) Psychiatric system survivors and emancipatory research: issues, overlaps and differences. In: Barnes C, Mercer G, eds. *Doing Disability Research*. Disability Press, Leeds

Beard JC (1995) *Illicit Drug Use: Acute and Chronic Pharmacological Intervention*. Quay Books, Mark Allen Publishing Ltd, Wiltshire

Becker H, Mainman L (1975) Socio-behavioral determinants of compliance with health and medical care. *Recom Med Care* **13**: 10–24 (cited by McKie, 1994)

Becker C (1991) *Living and Relating: An Introduction to Phenomenology*. Sage, London

Bee H (1985) *The Developing Child*. Harper and Row, USA

Bell A, Weinberg M (1978) *Homosexualities: A Study of Diversity Amongst Men and Women*. Simon and Schuster, New York

Benedek T (1938) Adaptation to reality in early infancy. *Psychoanal Q* **7**: 200–15

Bernstein GA (1998) *Anxiety and Depression Linked to Physical Symptoms in Teens*. The Australian Academy of Child and Adolescent Psychology Homepage: http://www.aacap.org

Bernstein GA (1997) *Somatic Symptoms in Anxious-Depressed School Refusers*. TAACAP, e-mail: mrscott@aacap.org. Homepage: http://www.aacap.org

Blanche HT, Parkes M (1997) Christianity. In: Parkes M, Laungani P, Young B, eds. *Death and Bereavement Across Cultures*. Routledge, London

Blumenthal S, Kupfer D (1990) *Suicide over the Life Cycle: Risk Factors, Assessment and Treatment of Suicide Patients*. American Academic Press, Washington

Bolton I (1987) *My Son — My Son*. Bolton Press, USA

Bowlby J (1979) *The Making and Breaking of Affection Bonds*. Tavistock/Routledge, London

Boyle C (1991) *The Employment Question: Will There be a Return to Full Employment*? University of Central England, Birmingham

Boyle C (1998) *After Work: a personal view by Connell Boyle*. BBC Community Programme Unit, London: e-mail: cpu@bbc.co.uk

Bradshaw A (1996) Does science need religion. In: Farmer E, ed. *Exploring the Spiritual Dimension of Care*. Quay Books, Mark Allen Publishing Ltd, Wiltshire

Bradshaw J (1965) *Home Coming*. Piatkus, USA

Breakwell G (1996) *Coping with Threatened Identities*. Methuen, London

Briere J, Conte J (1993) Self-reported amnesia for abuse in adults molested as children. *J Traum Stress* **6**(1): 21–31

Brown GW, Harris T (1978) *Social Origins of Depression*. Tavistock, London

Brown R, Kulik J (1977) Flashbulb memories. *Cognition* **5**: 73–99

Burleson BR, Albrecht TL, Goldsmith DJ, Sarason I (1994) *The Communication of Social Support: Messages, Interactions, Relationships and Community*. Sage, London

Burlington D, Freud A (1944) *Infants without Families*. George Allen and Unwin, London

Burt C (1969) *The Young Delinquent*. University of London Press, London

Citizens Income Study Centre (1998) *Citizens Income Newsletter*. London: e-mail: www.citizens-income.org.uk

Coles R (1989) *The Call of Stories*. Houghton Mifflin, Maryland

Conant JB (1962) Social dynamite in our larger cities. *Crime Delin* **8**: 102–5

Connell PH (1965) Suicidal attempts in childhood and adolescence. In: Howell SJ, ed. *Modern Perspectives in Child Psychiatry*. Oliver & Boyd, Edinburgh

Conway MA (1990a) *Autobiographic Memory: An Introduction*. Open University Press, Milton Keynes

Crain WC (1980) *Theories of Development: Concepts and Applications*. Prentice Hall, Englewood Cliffs, USA

Crook MH (1992) *Please Listen to Me*. International Self-Counselling Press, Canada

Csikszentmihalyi M, Larson R (1984) *Being Adolescent: Conflict and Growth in the Teenage Years*. Basic Books, New York

Dale PN (1985) *Many Mansions: The Growth of Religion in Bolton: 1750–1850*. Kwickprint, Bolton

Dennis J, Draper P, Holland S *et al* (1982) *Health Promotion in the Reorganised NHS*. The Health Services, 26 Nov (cited by Mackintosh, 1996)

Department of Health (1992) *The Health of the Nation: A Strategy for Health*. HMSO, London

Dominian J (1990) *Depression*. Wm Collins and Sons, Glasgow

Douglas J (1989) *Behaviour Problems in Young Children*. Tavistock, London

Duck S (1994) *Meaningful Relationships*. Sage, London

Durkheim E (1952) *Suicide* (trans Spaulding J, Simpson G). Routledge and Kegan Paul Ltd, London

Dyregrow A, Kingsley J (1991) *Grief in Children: A Handbook for the Professionals*. Jessica Kingsley, London

Early E (1993) *The Raven's Return: The Influence of Post Traumatic Disorder on Individuals and Culture*. Chiron, New York

Edmonds J (1990) *The Impact of Suicide. Lifeline*. The Newsletter of the National Association of Bereavement Services (NABS), London

Elkind D (1981) *The Hurried Child: Growing up Too Fast*. Addison-Wesley, Reading, MA

Erikson EH (1950) *Childhood and Society*. Norton and Co, New York

Erikson EH (1976) Borgs life cycle. *Daedalus* **105**: 1–28

Fanu R (1998) *Humor and Stress Humor home page*: Webspinner: Lois Richter: e-mail: LRichter@mother.com

Farmer P (1998) *The Samaritans and Young People*. The Samaritans, Slough

Featherstone M (1991) *Consumer Culture and Postmodernism*. Sage, London (cited by Nettleton, 1995)

Festinger L (1957) *A Theory of Cognitive Dissonance*. Stanford University Press, Stanford

Finney A (1998) When death haunts the track. *The Independent* 12 December (cited by Wertheimer, 1991)

Fishbein M (1967) Attitude and the prediction of behavior. In: Fishbein M, ed. *Readings in Attitude, Theory and Measurement*. J Wiley and Sons, New York

Fitzgerald H (1992) *The Grieving Child: A Parent's Guide*. Simon and Schuster, New York

Foy DW (1992) *Treating PTSD: Cognitive Strategies*. Guildford Press, USA

Frommer EA (1968) Depressive illness in childhood. In: Coppen A, Walk RM, eds. *Recent Developments in Affective Disorders*. RMPA, London (as cited by Dominion, 1990)

Frosh S (1991) *Identity Crisis: Modernity, Psychoanalysis and the Self*. Macmillan, London

Fulton R (1995) The contemporary funeral: Functional or dysfunctional? In: Wass H, Niemeyer RA, eds: *Dying: Facing the Facts*. Taylor and Frances, London

Giddens A (1991) *Modernity and Self Identity: Self and Society in the Late Modern Age*. Polity, Cambridge

Gilbert P (1992) *The Evolution of Powerlessness*. Lawrence Erhaum Associates, London

Global Ideas Bank (1998) *The Psychology of Happiness*. email: rhino@dial.pipex.com; home page: http://www.newciv.org/GIB/

Goodwin J (1987) *The Aetiology of Combat Related Post Traumatic Stress Disorder*. American Psychological Association. http:www.traum-pages.com

Gould RL (1978) *Transformations: Growth and Change in Adult Life*. Simon and Schuster, New York

Gorer G (1965) *Death, Grieving and Mourning in Contemporary Britain*. Cesset, London

Hahn J (1998) How to identify people at risk of committing suicide. *The Morning News of NWA Online*

Hemmings P (1995) Communicating with children through play. In: Smith SC, Pennells M, eds. *Interventions with Bereaved Children*. Jessica Kingsley, London

Hersh RH, Miller TP, Fielding GD (1980) *Models of Moral Education: An Appraisal*. Longman Group, New York

Hetrick ES, Martin AD (1987) Developmental issues and their resolution for gay and lesbian adolescents. *J Homosexuality* **14**(1/2): 25– 43 (cited by Markowe LA, 1997)

Higgins R (1993) Hate in nursery rhymes: captive audience, essential message. In: Varma V, ed. *How and Why Children Hate*. Jessica Kingsley, London

Holland S (1975) Adolescence and Politics: The student revolution. In: Meyerson S, ed. *Adolescence: The Crisis of Adjustment: A Study of Adolescence by the Tavistock Clinic and other British Experts*. Allen and Unwin, London

Hollinger P (1978) Epidemiological issues in youth suicide. In: Pfeffer C, ed. *Suicide among Youth*. American Psychiatric Press, USA

Hunt W, Robbins I (1998) Telling stories of the war: aging war veterans coping with their memories through narrative. Oral history. *J Oral History Society* **26**(2): 57–64

Hutchinson SA, Wilson HS (1994) The benefits of participating in research interviews. *J Nurs Scholarship* **26**(2): 161–4

Ingeldrew D (1989) Target setting the health of populations: some observations. *Health Prom Int* **4**(1): 357–69

Jackson J, Walker J, Jones B (1988) *Moon Walker*. Culver Studios, USA

Jamison KR (1996) Manic depressive illness and creativity. *Scientific American: Mysteries of the Mind* (special issue) March 1996: 44–9

Jenkins RA, Cavanaugh JC (1985) Examining the relationship between the development of the concept of death and overall development. *Omega* **16**: 193–9

Kastenbaum RJ (1967) *The Child's Understanding of Death: How does it Develop*? Beacon, Boston

Kastenbaum RJ (1981) *Death, Society and Human Experience*. Mosby, London

Kastenbaum RJ (1986) Death in the world of adolescence. In: Corr AC, McNeil MC, eds. *Adolescence and Death*. Springer Publishing, New York

Kenny C (1994) *Cotton Everywhere: Recollections of Northern Women Textile Workers*. Aurora Press, Bolton

Kenny C (1998a) *A Northern Thanatology*. Quay Books, Mark Allen Publishing Ltd, Wiltshire

Kenny C (1998b) *A Thanatology of War*. Quay Books, Mark Allen Publishing Ltd, Wiltshire

Kenny C (1998c) *A Thanatology of the Child*. Quay Books, Mark Allen Publishing Ltd, Wiltshire

Kitzinger S, Kitzinger C (1989) *Talking with Children about Things that Matter*. Pandora, London

Klein M (1960) *Our Adult World and its Roots in Infancy.* Tavistock, London

Kobler AL, Stotland E (1964) *The End of Hope*. Macmillan, London

Kohlberg L (1970) *The Child as a Moral Philosopher: Readings in Developmental Psychology Today.* CRM Books, Del Mar, CA

Kourany RFC (1987) Suicide among homosexual adolescents. *J Homosexuality* **13**(4): 111–17 (cited by Markowe, 1997)

Kubler-Ross E (1983) *On Children and Death*. Macmillan, New York

Kranzler EM (1990) Early childhood bereavement. *J Am Acad Child Adolesc* **29**: 514–20

Krystal JH (1987) *Integration and Self-healing after Trauma Alexhymia: Psychoanalytic Reforms*. Analytic Press, New York

Lake T (1984) *Living with Grief.* Sheldon Press, SPCK, UK

Leenaars AA (1995) Suicide. In: Wass H, Neimeyer RA, eds. *Dying: Facing the Facts*. Taylor and Frances, London

Lendrum S, Syme G (1992) *The Gift of Tears: A Practical Approach to Loss and Bereavement Counselling*. Routledge, London

Levi (1986) *The Drowned and the Saved.* Penguin, London

Liften RJ (1973) *The Life of the Self.* Simon and Schuster, New York

Lourie RS (1957) Suicide and attempted suicide in children and adolescents. *Texas Med* 58–68 (cited by Dominian, 1990)

Lukas C, Seiden H (1987) *Silent Grief: Living in the Wake of Suicide*. Macmillan, London (cited by Wertheimer, 1991)

Mackintosh N (1996) *Promoting Health: An Issue for Nurses*. Quay Books, Mark Allen Publishing Limited, Wiltshire

Manninger K (1938) *Man Against Himself.* Harcourt Brace, New York

Markowe LA (1997) *Redefining the Self: Coming Out as a Lesbian*. Polity Press, Cambridge

Mc Clure GMG (1984) Recent trends in suicide amongst the young. *Br J Psychiatry* (as cited by Dominion, 1990)

Mc Kie L (1994) *Risky Behaviours and Healthy Lifestyles*. Quay Books, Mark Allen Publishing Ltd, Wiltshire

Mercy J (1997) *The Epidemiology and Prevention of Suicide*. The University of Queensland, Young People at Risk Programme, Royal Brisbane Hospital, Herston, QLD4029, Fax: 61733655466: Tel: 61733655457

Miell D, Dallos R (1996) *Social Interactions and Personal Relationships*. Sage, London

Milligan S, Clare A (1993) *Depression and How to Survive It.* Ebury Press, London

Montessori M (1917) *The Advanced Montessori Method (Vol. 1) Spontaneous Activity in Education* (F Simmonds trans). Robert Bentley, Cambridge

Murry H (1967) Death to the world: The passion of Herman Melvill. In: Shneidman E, ed. *Essays on Self-Destruction*. Science House, New York

Myers DG, Diener ED (1996) The pursuit of happiness. *Scientific American: Mysteries of the Mind* (special edition) March: 40–44

Nagy M (1959) The child's view of death. In: Fiefel H, ed. *The Meaning of Death*. McGraw Hill, New York

Naidoo J, Wills J (1994) *Health Promotion: Foundations for Practice*. Ballière Tindall, London

Nettleton S (1995) *The Sociology of Health and Illness*. Polity Press, Cambridge

Oakley A (1991) Interviewing women: A contradiction in terms. In: Roberts H, ed. *Doing Feminist Research*. Routledge, London

O'Connell WE (1995) *Humor: An Antidote for Stress*. Humor Home Page: Webspinner: Lois Richter e-mail: LRichter@mother.com

Otto U (1972) Suicide acts by children and adolescents. *Acta Psychiatr Scand* **233**(suppl) (as cited by Dominion, 1990)

University of Queensland (1998) *Suicide and Young People*. University of Queensland, Young people at Risk Program, Royal Brisbane Hospital, Herston, QLD4029

Ussher J (1991) *Women's Madness: Misogyny or Mental Illness*. Harvester Wheatsheaf, Hertfordshire

Parkes C *et al* (1997) *Death and Bereavement across Cultures*. Routledge, London

Pasho M (1998) *Differences between Younger and Older Child Suicides Analyzed*. (TAACAP fact sheet) email: mrscott@aacap.org Homepage: http://www.aacap.org

Pepper D (1996) *Modern Environmentalism: An Introduction*. Routledge, London

Piaget J (1932) *The Moral Judgment of the Child*. Macmillan, New York

Piaget J (1965) *The Child's Conception of the World*. Littlefield Adams, Ottowa NT

Plummer K (1995) *Telling Sexual Stories: Power, Change and Social Worlds* . Routledge, London (cited by Markowe, LA, 1997)

Rioch S (1994) *Suicidal Children and Adolescents: Crisis and Preventative Care*. Celia Publications, Durham

Riochlin G (1967) How younger children view death and themselves. In: Grollman BA, ed. *Explaining Death to Children*. Beacon Press, Boston

Rosenberg M, Eddy D, Wolpert R, Broumas E (1989) Developing strategies to prevent youth suicide. In: Pfeffer C, ed. *Suicide Among Youth*. American Psychiatric Press, USA

Rotter JB, Chance J, Phares EJ, eds (1972) *Applications of a Social Learning Theory of Personality Development*. Holt, Reinhart and Winston, New York

Rowan J (1983) *The Reality Game: A Guide to Humanistic Counselling and Therapy*. Routledge. London

Royal College of Psychiatrists (1998a) *Surviving Adolescence*. Internet publication: Website: http://www.demon.co.uk//repsych e-mail:repsych@repsych.ac.uk

Royal College of Psychiatrists (1998b) *Teen Suicide Fact Sheet*. Internet publication. Website: http://www.demon.co.uk//repsych: e-mail: repsych@repsych.ac.uk

Saigh PA (1992) *Post Traumatic Stress Disorder: A Behavioural Approach to Assessment and Treatment*. Pergamon Press, Oxford

Samaritans (1998a) *Suicide Fact sheet*. The Samaritans, London

Segal L (1997) Sexualities. In: Woodward K, ed. *Identity and Difference: Culture, Media and Identities*. Sage, London

Seligman MEP (1975) *On Depression, Development and Death*. WH Freeman, San Francisco

Shakespeare T (1996) Disability, identity and difference. In: Barnes C, Mercer G, eds. *Exploring the Divide: Illness and Disability*. The Disability Press, University of Leeds, Leeds

Shaton CP (1973) Stress disorders amongst Vietnam combat veterans self-help movement. *Am J Orthopsych* **43**(4): 43–53

Shneidman E (1963) Orientations towards suicide. In: White R, ed. *The Study of Lives*. Atherton, New York (cited by Leenaars, 1995)

Shneidman E (1973) Suicide. In: *Encyclopedia Britannica*. William Benton, Chicago: 383–5

Shneidman E (1985) *Definition of Suicide*. J Wiley and Sons, New York (cited by Leenaars, 1995)

Smart B (1992) *Modern Conditions, Postmodern Controversies*. Routledge, London (cited by Nettleton, 1995)

Spitz RA and Wolfe (1946) *Anaclitic Depression: Psychoanalytic Studies of the Child*. Hogarth Press, London (cited by Dominian, 1990)

Squire LR (1994) Declarative and non-declarative memory: supporting learning and memory. In: Schacter DL, Tuluing J, eds. *Memory Systems*. MIT Press, Cambridge MA

Stack S (1991) Social correlates of suicide by age: Media impacts. In: Leenaars A, ed. *Life Span Perspectives in Suicide*. Plenum, New York

Stanley L (1994) Thoughts on Cotton Everywhere. In: Kenny C. *Cotton Everywhere*. Aurora, Bolton

Stengel E (1964) *Suicide and Attempted Suicide*. Macgibbon and Kee, England

Sugerman L (1986) *Life Span Development: Concepts, Theories and Interventions*. Routledge, London

Sutherland S (1998) *Breakdown: A Personal Crisis and a Medical Dilemma*. Open University Press, Milton Keynes

Tajfel H, ed (1978) *Differentiation Between Groups: Studies in the Social Psychology of Intergroup Relationships*. Academic Press, London

Talley JH (1998) *Questions and Answers About Major Depression*. Thomas A Arsenault's home page: Website: http://.winternet.com/~taa/ e-mail: (winternet) taa@winternet.com

The Compassionate Friends (1993a) *To Bereaved Grandparents*. TCF, Bristol

The Compassionate Friends (1993b) *Helping Younger Bereaved Brothers and Sisters*. TCF, Bristol

The Compassionate Friends (1993c) *Grieving Couples*. TCF, Bristol

The Compassionate Friends (1998a) *Introducing the Compassionate Friends*. TCF, Bristol

The Compassionate Friends (1998b) *After Suicide*. TCF, Bristol

The Compassionate Friends (1998c) *No Death so Sad*. TCF, Bristol

Van Kolk BA, Blitz R, Burr WA, Hartman E (1984) Nightmares and trauma: lifelong and traumatic memories in veterans. *Am J Psychiatry* **141**: 187–90

Wallston, KA, Wallston BS (1978) Health locus of control. *Health Educ Monogr* **6**: 2

Wass H (1995) Death in the Lives of Children and Adolescents. In: Wass H, Niemeyer RA, eds. *Dying: Facing the Facts*.Taylor and Frances, London

Wass H, Miller MD, Stevenson RG (1989) Factors affecting adolescent behavior and attitudes towards destructive rock lyrics. *Death Studies* **13**: 287–303

Watt NE, Nicholi A (1979) Early death of a parent as an etiological factor in schizophrenia. *Am J Orthopsych* **49**: 465–73

Weinstein J (1998) A proper haunting: the need in mourning to maintain a continuing relationship with the dead. *J Social Work Pract* **12**(1): 93–102

Wertheimer A (1991) *A Special Scar: The Experience of People Bereaved by Suicide*. Routledge/Tavistock, London

Whitehead M (1987) The Health Divide. In: Townsend P, Davidson N, Whitehead N, eds. *Inequalities in Health*. Penguin, Harmondsworth

Whitworth SK, Wienstock CS (1979) *Adult Development: The Differentiation of Experience*. Holt, Reinholt and Winston, New York

Woodward K (1997) *Identity and Difference: Culture, Media and Identities*. Sage, London

Wooten I (1998) *Humor, Stress and Depression*. Humor home page: Webspinner:Lois Richer e-mail:LRichter@mother.com

Wright B (1993) *Caring in Crisis*. Churchill Livingston, Edinburgh

Wrobeski A (1991) *Suicide Survivors*. Afterwards Publishing, USA

Youth Crisis (1998) *Warning Signs of Suicide*. Youth Crisis Stabilization Program, Community Health and Counselling Service, Bangor, Maine

Index

D

E

F

G

N

O

P

T

U

V

W

Y